P9-CLR-655

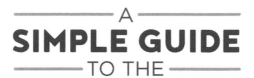

A
SIMPLE GUIDE
TO THE

PALEO
AUTOIMMUNE
PROTOCOL

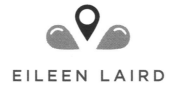

EILEEN LAIRD

Copyright © 2015 Eileen Laird

Phoenixhelix.com

All rights reserved. No part of this book may be used or
reproduced in any manner whatsoever without written
permission except in the case of brief quotations embodied
in critical articles and reviews.

Acknowledgement: The author writes a regular column for
Paleo Magazine, called "Autoimmune Answers." Versions
of Chapters 14, 15 and 17 first appeared as part of that
series. Reprinted here with permission. To subscribe, visit
Paleomagonline.com.

Disclaimer: The reader understands that the author is not
a medical professional. The information included in this
book is for inspirational and educational purposes only. It
is not intended nor implied to be a substitute for professional
medical advice. The reader should always consult his or her
healthcare provider to determine the appropriateness of the
information for their own situation. The author is not liable
for any loss or damage allegedly arising from the information
presented in this book.

Cover & Interior Design by Chelsey Luther
AIP Food Pyramid Illustration by Eileen Laird
Phoenix Illustration by Beny Noveva

This book is dedicated to anyone whose
autoimmune disease knocked them down so hard,
they wondered if they would ever rise again.

Never underestimate your ability to rise.
We all have a phoenix within us.

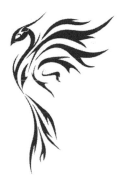

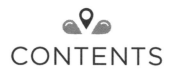

CONTENTS

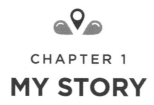

CHAPTER 1

MY STORY

I was a 43-year old healthy woman, working full-time as a massage therapist, and hiking the mountains on the weekends for fun. Then one morning, I awoke to a swollen joint on the bottom of my foot, and it hurt to put on my shoes. I thought, "Well, that's weird," and just assumed the feeling would pass. Little did I know that pain would spread across the balls of both feet, then to my hands, then ricochet around my body like Flare Russian Roulette. Within six months, I couldn't walk without limping; I couldn't open a jar or lift a pan or raise my arms over my head. Each morning I'd rise from bed feeling like I was 90 years old; each night a joint would flare so extremely I would have to immobilize it to keep from gasping and crying from the pain. If it was my wrist, it went into a brace; if it was my shoulder, it went into a sling; if it was my knee, I had to get off my feet the rest of the night; and if it was my jaw, I couldn't open my mouth to speak or to eat. Rheumatoid arthritis had laid claim to my body and my life. In the 43 years prior, I thought I knew what pain was; I had no clue.

I was terrified. I had worked with clients with autoimmune disease. I knew there was no cure. I knew the lifelong medications came with serious side effects and often didn't work at all. I desperately wanted another solution, and Google led me to Paleo. I remember telling my mother I was going to try to heal through diet, and she literally laughed out loud. She had seen advertisements on TV that made the medications look like miracles. She was raised to believe pills provided the cure, and food had nothing to do with our health (or lack thereof). She's not alone; that's the mainstream perspective. But once you step outside of the processed-food-marketing bubble, it makes sense that what we put in our bodies all day every day has a huge impact on how we feel. The trick is figuring out which foods harm us and which foods lead to healing. Taking out the processed foods is a no-brainer, but what about the rest? I did a few experiments on my own, trying vegetarianism and veganism, but my inflammation continued to skyrocket. It wasn't until I began a nutrient-dense paleo diet that my inflammation started to lower instead.

I'm not an overnight success story. Instead, it was a year of slow and steady improvements. My flares went from daily occurrences, to every few days, to every few weeks, to every few months, to eventually disappearing altogether. I slowly went from feeling exhausted, to feeling a low pulse of energy, to feeling like I had energy to burn. I regained my ability to exercise, first doing gentle stretching, then 15 minutes on an exercise bike, then walking one mile, then two, then returning to the mountain hikes I love. I went back to work part-time, then full-time, and did a brief period of working overtime because I was so excited to be able to work again. (But that's not healthy either—more on that later in the book.) So, I'm back to working just full-time now.

I'm not 100% cured; I still have rheumatoid arthritis. But I was able to reduce my symptoms by 95%. For me, that's the difference between a life of disability and a full and beautiful life. I reclaimed not only my health, but my joy. The inflammation that now remains in my body is a whisper, where it used to be a scream. I'm so grateful that food can be medicine. And I'm not alone.

CHAPTER 2

WHAT DOES REVERSING AUTOIMMUNE DISEASE MEAN?

Let's be honest, we all want a cure. We want to kick our autoimmune disease to the curb and leave it behind us, never to affect our lives again. Unfortunately, when it comes to autoimmune disease, once that switch is flipped in our body, it's part of who we are. But don't close the book! It doesn't mean we can't take control of our health and feel exponentially better. The normal course of autoimmune disease is that we have a lifetime of worsening symptoms and loss of abilities. The outlook is bleak. Reversing autoimmune disease is about reversing that process. By changing your diet and lifestyle, your symptoms start to improve and you regain abilities you thought were lost forever. It's incredibly empowering and definitely worth the effort.

What does this look like? You read my story; that's one example. Here are some others:

- **Robyn Latimer has Lupus.** At her worst, she was hospitalized for two weeks with a life-threatening flare. She was then put on steroid and immunosuppressant medication and took 36 pills a day for years, yet she still had autoimmune symptoms: fatigue, brain fog, joint pain, and bodywide stiffness. After two weeks of switching to the paleo diet, she was 100% symptom-free. She's now off all her medications and has been in remission for over three years.

- **Mickey Trescott has Celiac and Hashimoto's.** At her worst, she experienced anxiety, insomnia, depression, exhaustion, hair loss, joint pain, dizziness, brain fog, neuropathy, and anemia, along with severe hormone, blood sugar and blood pressure imbalances. She lost her ability to work and lost faith she would ever get well. Thyroid medication alone didn't reverse her symptoms, nor did simply going gluten-free. The key for her was the paleo autoimmune protocol (AIP). After two years following the AIP, she works full time and has the energy to live on a sustainable farmstead with her husband. She's symptom-free, strong enough to do heavy labor, and has a vibrant, happy outlook on life again.

- **Whitney Ross-Gray has Multiple Sclerosis.** She once said, "I'd rather have MS than give up bread." When she started to lose her ability to walk, she changed her mind and changed her diet. At her worst, she experienced vision loss, leg weakness, brain fog, fatigue, bladder control issues, and sexual dysfunction. Now she is 95% symptom-free and has been able to avoid all medication.

- **Martine Partridge has Crohns.** When she was 17 years old, she had a flare so extreme that her weight plummeted to 75 pounds, she was hospitalized with life-threatening complications, and the doctors recommended a complete removal of her colon. Her family took her home against medical advice and started her on a healing diet along with numerous medications. Now, 20 years later, she still has her colon and her health. She's not medication-free, but she has been able to reduce her medication substantially, and the combination of diet, lifestyle and medication allow her to enjoy a high quality of life.

- **Shannon Keating has Psoriasis.** It first appeared on her stomach and quickly spread bodywide to her arms, legs, chest, back and face. She was actually paleo at the time, and it wasn't until she transitioned to the AIP that the psoriasis went away. Within two weeks, she started to notice improvement. Within two months, 75% of the spots were gone. A year later, all of the spots are gone, with just a few small scars on her legs reminding her that she ever had psoriasis.

I could literally write a book of healing stories like these. Thousands of people are using the paleo autoimmune protocol to transform their lives. Some people achieve complete remission like Shannon and Robyn. Others are able to eliminate 95% of their symptoms and avoid the strong prescriptions, like Whitney. Others are able to dramatically lower their medication and improve their symptoms at the same time, like Martine and Mickey.

There are over 100 autoimmune diseases, so yours might not have been mentioned in the examples above. There's something I want you to know: autoimmune diseases have more in common than not. The process is the same no matter what your diagnosis—the immune system has lost the ability to discern self from non-self, and in its desire to protect us from something harmful, it accidentally attacks us instead. Our diagnosis is based on where that attack takes place. If it's your thyroid, it might be Hashimoto's or Graves' disease. If it's your joints, is might be rheumatoid arthritis or ankylosing spondylitis. If it's your digestive system, it might be Crohn's or ulcerative colitis. But in all those cases, and the other 100+ autoimmune diagnoses, the process is the same, and the AIP is a method for reversing that process. It's an anti-inflammatory, nutrient-dense diet that helps calm down our overstimulated immune system and rebuild our health from a cellular level.

This is the power of Epigenetics. Many of us were taught in school that we are a product of our genes, but science has advanced since our childhood. Researchers discovered that genes play only a small role in our health. Many healthy people are walking around with genes for diseases they don't have. How is that possible? Other factors—like diet and lifestyle—determine which genes get turned on. A cascade of events happens to trigger autoimmune disease in the body. The paleo autoimmune protocol is designed to reverse that cascade and slowly turn those genes off again. How cool is that?

CHAPTER 3

WHAT TO EXPECT FROM THIS BOOK

This guide is designed to be written like a conversation between friends, where I share the essential information you need to get started, in a book small enough to throw in your purse or backpack and carry with you. I know a lot of you just starting this journey are dealing with brain fog. I made this book easy to read and reference for that reason. It's a quick gateway to living the AIP life.

While this book is designed to be a quick guide, it's also designed to cover all the bases. You'll learn which foods you need to avoid, and which you should add to your diet. It includes grocery lists, meal planning tips, and advice for traveling and eating out at restaurants. We'll talk about navigating holiday traditions, getting support from family and friends, and what lifestyle interventions can make a big difference. I'll also teach you the food reintroduction process, which you start once you've seen a clear improvement in your autoimmune symptoms. Lastly, I'll share troubleshooting tips if you aren't seeing the improvement you seek.

What you won't find in this book are recipes, meal plans, or detailed scientific explanations. Why? Two reasons: (1) The book would be a multi-volume encyclopedia if I tried to include everything. (2) There are some wonderful AIP cookbooks and meal plans out there already, and more being published all the time. As for the science, Sarah Ballantyne has covered that in detail in *The Paleo Approach*.

The resource that's missing—and is greatly needed—is a simple guide. That's why I've written this one.

I'll be sharing a list of other AIP resources at the end of this book. I'll direct you to recipe archives online that are free, as well as cookbooks and meal plans that you can buy. I'll also include information about online support groups, group coaching classes, 1:1 consultants, and more. This is exciting because when I first started the AIP, there were no published resources and very little information online. The AIP is much easier to follow now because so much more support is available. This community is growing larger all the time. We are changing the definition of living with autoimmune disease. I hope you'll join us!

CHAPTER 4

WHAT IS THE PALEO AUTOIMMUNE PROTOCOL (THE AIP)?

The AIP is a diet and lifestyle program designed to reduce inflammation, heal digestion, deliver nutrition that supports health, and ultimately reverse autoimmune disease. There are four elements to the protocol, and I'll discuss all of them in detail later in the book. Here's a quick overview.

1. **Foods to Avoid.** These are foods that have the potential to increase inflammation, stimulate the immune system, and/or irritate the digestive tract. The main categories are processed foods, additives, refined oils, refined sugars, grains, legumes, dairy, nightshades, eggs, nuts, seeds and alcohol.

2. **Foods to Eat.** Not all foods are created equal. You've heard of empty calories. Well, the opposite of that are nutrient-dense calories, and they're the foods you seek out on the AIP. The more nutrients we provide our bodies,

the more building blocks they have to heal. These healing foods include wild-caught seafood, grass-fed meats,
organ meats, healthy fats, fermented foods, bone broth,
and a wide variety of vegetables.

3. **Food Reintroductions.** When it comes to food, the
AIP has an elimination phase and a reintroduction phase.
Many people make the mistake of thinking the elimination phase lasts forever. It doesn't. When you see clear
improvement in your autoimmune symptoms, you can
begin a careful reintroduction process where you test each
food to see how your body reacts. This is how you personalize the AIP for you. I'll guide you through this process
later in the book.

4. **Lifestyle Choices.** It might surprise you to learn that
poor lifestyle choices can cause autoimmune flares, just
as much as poor dietary choices. Your diet can be perfect,
but if you're living a high-stress life and sacrificing sleep,
that's a recipe for illness. The AIP is a holistic approach to
healing, and it includes stress management, prioritizing
sleep, healthy movement, time outdoors, making time
for joy, getting support when we need it, and sometimes
making tough choices to remove stress from our lives.

CHAPTER 5

FOODS TO AVOID AND WHY

The AIP starts with the paleo diet, removing foods that are problematic for human beings in general. It's based on the simple premise that our bodies weren't designed to eat modern foods, which is why we have an epidemic of chronic disease. Returning to a hunter-gatherer style of eating will also return us to health:

FOODS TO AVOID ON THE PALEO DIET
Processed Food—Anything Artificial
Refined Sugars
Refined Vegetable Oils
Grains (including corn)
Dried Legumes (including soy and peanuts)
Dairy (optional)

Avoiding processed food is a no-brainer. We all know that if we can't pronounce the ingredient list on a food label, then it's not good for our health. Here's a second thing to consider: most foods that are shelf-stable—meaning they can sit on a grocery store shelf and *not* rot—aren't food the way nature intended. This naturally makes them difficult for our bodies to digest. Even packaged foods with ingredients that sound natural aren't natural at all. They're engineered foods. In other words, processed foods you find in the "health food store" are still foods to avoid.

I also don't think it will surprise you to learn that sugar is bad for our health, and most people eat far too much. But you might be shocked to realize just how much: In 1822, the average American ate less than two teaspoons of sugar daily. In 2012, the average American ate 31 teaspoons of sugar daily, and my guess is that most didn't realize it. Americans rely on restaurant food and packaged foods as a major part of their diet, and sugar is added to almost all of them.

When it comes to oils, avoid margarine (of course), but also canola, corn, cottonseed, flax seed, grape seed, peanut, safflower, soybean and sunflower oils. Although many of these have been marketed to us as "healthy" oils, the opposite is true. They're heavily processed, using heat, pressure and chemicals to extract the oils. The result is an unstable oil that goes rancid easily. Since all odor has been removed during processing, you can't tell that it's rancid. They're also high in omega-6 fatty acids (which increase inflammation). Canola oil is the only one marketed as high in omega-3 fatty acids (which are anti-inflammatory). However, canola comes from a toxic plant called rapeseed and has to go through heavy processing to remove the toxic compounds. The result isn't healthy.

What's the problem with grains? They're the base of the USDA food pyramid, and nutritionists have been telling us to increase our consumption for years, so it can be shocking to hear that they're bad for our health. Refined flours and grains have all of their nutrition stripped from them and convert quickly to sugar in the body. We've heard enough about gluten intolerance to understand why we need to avoid that. But what about other "whole grains"? Well, they contain anti-nutrients and enzyme inhibitors that make them hard to digest, and that means our bodies can't effectively absorb their nutrition. You've heard the phrase, "You are what you eat." Actually, "You are what you eat, digest and absorb." Whole grains also contain compounds that irritate the digestive tract and can cause leaky gut (a condition that coincides with and exacerbates autoimmunity). For more information on leaky gut, please read *The Paleo Approach*.

Dried legumes are the dried bean family: black beans, navy beans, kidney beans, soybeans, split peas, garbanzos, lentils, etc. They also include peanuts (misnamed as nuts). Dried legumes are similar to grains in that they also contain anti-nutrients and enzyme inhibitors, making them difficult to digest and increase inflammation in the body.

In the "Paleo Foods to Avoid" table at the start of this chapter, I put "optional" next to dairy, because it's a point of controversy in the paleo community. Strict paleo avoids all dairy for many reasons: Even raw dairy contains natural hormones that can affect hormone balance in human beings. Commercial milk contains even more. Dairy also contains lactose, a carbohydrate which many people around the world can't digest. It contains casein, a protein very similar in structure to gluten, which can cause similar health problems. It stimulates a histamine response which can mimic or exacerbate allergy and asthma symptoms. Those are a lot of reasons to avoid it, right? So, why is there any controversy? Well, some people find they tolerate *quality* dairy without any of those problems. By quality, I mean grass-fed, full-fat, raw dairy. In the paleo community, people who eat dairy in small amounts call themselves "Primal" as opposed to "Strict Paleo." On the autoimmune protocol, dairy is eliminated, and then reintroduced to test for tolerance.

ADDITIONAL FOODS TO AVOID ON THE AIP
Dairy (definitely)
Eggs
Nightshades (including nightshade spices)
Nuts
Seeds (including coffee and cocoa)
Alcohol
Emulsifiers and Thickeners
Stevia (and other non-nutritive sweeteners)
Fresh Legumes (green beans and green peas)
Fruit-Based and Seed-Based Spices
Nut-Based and Seed-Based Oils
Fruit is limited to a few pieces daily
Desserts only on special occasions

Don't panic—it's not forever! The foods in the above table are allowed on the paleo diet, but eliminated on the autoimmune protocol because they can potentially cause issues for many people with autoimmune disease. The difference is that these aren't avoided permanently. You eliminate these foods for a minimum of 30 days, and when you see clear improvement in your autoimmune symptoms, you follow a careful reintroduction process, where you learn which of these foods you tolerate and can add back into your diet. I'll guide you through this reintroduction process later in the book. First, let me introduce you to the people behind the AIP, and then I'll explain why these foods are temporarily eliminated.

Who created the autoimmune protocol? The AIP is the brainchild of Dr. Loren Cordain, a scientist who discovered that certain primal foods can sometimes trigger inflammation in people with autoimmune disease (dairy, eggs, nightshades, nuts, seeds and alcohol). Since then, another scientist, Dr. Sarah Ballantyne, delved into the research behind the protocol and expanded the AIP in her book *The Paleo Approach*. She added some extra eliminations: emulsifiers, stevia, fresh legumes, and a few other spices and oils. She wasn't trying to be mean! She believes these foods can be obstacles to autoimmune healing and tried to create the healthiest protocol possible.

I've already discussed dairy.

Let's talk about eggs. The natural purpose of an egg is to develop into a chicken. The yolk contains all the nutrition that baby chick would need to grow. The white is a defensive barrier against predators, and it's full of things that interfere with our digestion. Egg white has also been shown to be able to pass through the intestinal wall and set off an autoimmune response.

You may have heard of the term "deadly nightshade" referring to a plant called belladonna, which was used as a poison in ancient times. Lesser known are the commonly eaten vegetables in the same nightshade family. They aren't deadly, but they contain enough toxins to cause inflammation in some people, particularly those with autoimmune disease. In fact, for many of us, they're the strongest inflammatory food. Here's a list of common nightshades to avoid: tomatoes, tomatillos, potatoes, eggplants, peppers (bell peppers, banana peppers, chili peppers), red pepper seasonings (paprika, chili powder, cayenne, and store-bought spice blends including curry), pimentos, pepinos, tamarillos, goji berries, ashwagandha (an ayurvedic herb) and tobacco. In addition, read labels carefully. If you ever see unnamed "spices" or "natural flavors," it's often nightshades. Similar sounding foods that aren't nightshades: sweet potatoes and peppercorns (black, white, green and pink). Tip: some nightshade lists on the internet are inaccurate and list foods that aren't nightshades at all. If you ever wonder if a food is a nightshade, just look it up in Wikipedia. If it's in the Solanaceae family, it's a nightshade. If it's from another plant family, it's not. One more note: I thought it was crazy to give up nightshade spices—it's such a small amount; how could it matter? Trust me on this—it does. I gave up the vegetables but kept eating the spices, and my flares didn't stop until I gave up the spices too. This is a common story in the AIP community.

Nuts and seeds are eliminated because they can be difficult to digest. Most people with autoimmune disease have leaky gut, so it's wise to avoid foods that irritate the digestive tract. Two seeds that many of us love more than all others are coffee and cocoa. To help you with your chocolate cravings, carob is a similar-tasting substitute that is allowed on the AIP. As for coffee, many people switch to green tea or yerba mate, which both have some caffeine and are allowed in moderation. Or you can find herbal coffee substitutes online—just check ingredients carefully!

Mainstream media likes to tout the benefits of moderate alcohol consumption, but the truth is, **alcohol worsens leaky gut**, feeds pathogenic bacteria, and interferes with our ability to sleep without waking in the middle of the night (and poor sleep can cause autoimmune flares). For those reasons, we avoid it on the AIP. The one exception is cooking; since most of the alcohol burns off under heat, we can use grain-free alcohol in recipes.

Emulsifiers and thickeners include additives like guar gum, carrageenan, xanthum gum, cellulose gum and lecithin. They are common additives to things like canned coconut milk sold in stores. Unfortunately, they also irritate the digestive tract and cause leaky gut, which is why we avoid them on the AIP. There are two additive-free brands of coconut milk available: Aroy-D and Natural Value. You can also make your own coconut milk simply by blending hot water and shredded unsweetened coconut together at high speed and then straining. (Recipes are available online.)

It may surprise you to see stevia on the "avoid" list because it has been touted as a healthy alternative to sugar. The concern is that some stevia compounds have structures similar to hormones and can affect hormone balance (which in turn affects autoimmune expression). Other non-nutritive sweeteners include artificial ones like nutrasweet and saccharin, but also sugar alcohols like xylitol and sorbitol. There's a misperception that if they don't contain calories, they can't hurt us, but research shows they can negatively affect both digestion and metabolism. In *The Paleo Approach*, Ballantyne writes, "There is no way to cheat desserts." It's better to have natural sugars like honey and maple syrup (in moderation) on the AIP than non-nutritive sweeteners.

Earlier in this chapter, I talked about the problems with dried legumes. **Fresh legumes** are often eaten on a regular paleo diet since they don't have the digestive challenges of dried varieties. Because people with autoimmune disease are more sensitive, and our digestion is often compromised, Ballantyne recommends eliminating fresh legumes as well: green beans, snow peas, snap peas, and green peas. However, these are one of the first foods she recommends reintroducing, and most people reintroduce them successfully.

The same goes for **fruit and seed-based spices, and nut and seed-based oils.** Avoiding them is a recommendation to be on the safe side. Rather than listing all of the spices to avoid, Chapter 10 will list all of the ones you *can* eat, along with some AIP-friendly recommendations for ways to add flavor to your food. Food does *not* have to bland on the AIP, I promise.

The last thing to mention is the role of natural sugar on the AIP. I mentioned in the paragraph on stevia that small amounts of natural sugars are allowed on the AIP. When it comes to fruit, 1–3 servings per day is fine; just don't binge. As for desserts like cookies, cakes and ice creams, there are now lots of AIP-friendly recipes available, but they're designed to be eaten on special occasions. Too much sugar will derail your healing, even if it's natural. It doesn't mean you can never have a cookie, but it shouldn't be part of your daily diet.

You might be overwhelmed at the end of this chapter, thinking, *There's no way I can do this! This is too much!* Take a deep breath, and keep reading. The next chapter tells you all the foods you CAN eat, which is the joy of the AIP. The chapter after that gives you lots of advice for successfully making this protocol a part of your life. It is hard—you're right and I won't lie to you—but there are ways to make it easier, and I'm going to show you how.

SUMMARY OF FOODS TO AVOID

PALEO

Processed Food (anything artificial)

Refined Sugars

Refined Vegetable Oils

Grains (including corn)

Dried Legumes (including soy and peanuts)

Dairy (optional)

AIP

All of the Above Plus:

Dairy (definitely)

Eggs

Nightshades (including nightshade spices)

Nuts

Seeds (including coffee and cocoa)

Alcohol

Emulsifiers and Thickeners

Stevia (and other non-nutritive sweeteners)

Fresh Legumes (green beans and green peas)

Fruit-Based and Seed-based spices

Nut-Based and Seed-Based Oils

Fruit is limited to a few pieces daily

Desserts only on special occasions

CHAPTER 6

FOODS TO EAT AND WHY

Now we're at the good part: all the wonderful foods we can enjoy on the AIP!

FOODS TO ENJOY
All Meat, Poultry and Seafood
Healthy Fats
All Vegetables (except nightshades & legumes)
All Fruit (except goji berries which are a nightshade)
Natural Sweeteners (in moderation)
Coconut (in moderation)
Focus on nutrient-density & healing foods

When we change our diets and give up all of the foods we're accustomed to eating, it can feel like there's nothing left to eat. It's not true. I eat delicious food every day on the AIP, and you can too. You just need to open your mind to a different way of eating. You'll find new favorite foods, and soon it will feel both normal and delicious!

To begin, let's talk protein. Meat has been maligned for years, but it actually contains nutrition you can't find elsewhere. There's a reason many vegetarians become nutrient deficient, especially in the vital B vitamins. In fact, did you know that B12 deficiency can sometimes mimic autoimmune disease symptoms?

But what about the dangers of eating meat? According to Sarah Ballantyne, "Every study that looks at the correlation between meat consumption and cancer shows that correlation completely disappears as soon as they correct for vegetable consumption." Vegetables are a huge part of the AIP as well. As long as you eat both, it's a healthy diet.

What about meat quality? You want to choose the best that your budget allows. Your ideal choice is going to be grass-fed and organic. Conventional meat is less ideal. Here are some tips to get the best choices for your dollars:

- Seek budget cuts of the high-quality meat, like ground meats, stew meat, braising meats and organ meats. They're much less expensive than the steaks and tenderloins and also have a better nutrition profile.

- If you can only afford conventional meat, choose lean meats over fatty cuts because toxins are stored in the fat. (This isn't a concern with organic meats, since that fat is healthy.)

- Get to know your local grass-fed farmers. You can often buy directly from them at lower prices than the grocery store. Search: Localharvest.org.

What about the dangers of eating fish? With our oceans becoming more and more polluted, people are rightly concerned about mercury toxicity. Well, it turns out that seafood also contains selenium, and selenium acts protectively against mercury toxicity. As long as the fish contains more selenium than mercury, it's safe to eat. The vast majority of seafood fits this profile. The few exceptions are some of the largest fish like swordfish and shark. You want to avoid those.

What about fish quality? Again, you want to choose the best your budget allows. Your ideal choice is going to be wild-caught, sustainable, and high in omega-3 fatty acids (like salmon). Less ideal is farmed fish (like tilapia). Here are some seafood shopping tips:

- If you can't find quality fish locally, a great online source is Vital Choice Seafood: http://bit.ly/vitalseafood.
- Some of the fish richest in anti-inflammatory omega 3s are salmon, mackerel and sardines, all of which can be bought less expensively as canned fish. Just read labels carefully and choose ones without additives.
- Shop the sales and stock up on high-quality seafood when the price drops. It freezes and defrosts well.
- If you can only afford farmed fish, stick with the shellfish. They don't require any feed and are less prone to illness, so they have no need for medication.

So, that's your protein needs covered. **Let's talk about healthy fats.** Does that sound like an oxymoron? Having grown up in the "low-fat age," it can be shocking to learn that the science behind the low-fat recommendation was never sound. In fact, as Americans started eating less fat, chronic disease of all kinds skyrocketed. Our bodies need fat. Every cell membrane is made of 50% fat, and 60% of our brain is fat. Fats are the building blocks of our hormones, and many vitamins are fat-soluble, meaning we can't absorb them without fat. So, incorporate autoimmune-friendly fats into every meal. These include: coconut oil, lard, tallow, duck fat, red palm oil, extra virgin olive oil and avocado oil.

I mentioned above that vegetables are a big part of the AIP. They're actually the foundation of the diet. Terry Wahls recommends that we eat 6–9 cups vegetables daily. Sarah Ballantyne recommends we eat even more: 8–14 cups. Does that sound crazy to you? There's science behind these recommendations. Terry Wahls is the author of *The Wahls Protocol*. She's a physician with multiple sclerosis, who went from a wheelchair to a bicycle, by following a paleo diet that focused on the healing nutrition of vegetables. Vegetables contain micronutrients not found elsewhere, and the more variety we eat, the deeper our nutrition. Hunter-gatherers ate an average of 200 species of plants and animals each year. (That can be a fun goal to set for yourself!) Another benefit of consuming vegetables is that they contain fiber that feed the beneficial bacteria in our guts. Eat a combination of cooked and raw vegetables, for optimal nutrition. However, if you have digestive problems, cooked vegetables are easier to digest.

So, how do you eat that many veggies? I have some tips:
- First, those measurements are raw vegetables, and many vegetables shrink when cooked, especially greens.

- Second, take into account your body size. 6 cups is about right for a petite woman. 14 cups is suitable for a large man.
- Third, prioritize vegetables over snacks. Don't say you don't have room for vegetables if you have room for dessert.
- Fourth, smoothies are one way to increase vegetable intake, but be sure to drink them alongside a meal, to avoid blood sugar spikes.

What about fruit? It's absolutely allowed on the AIP, and when you stop eating sugar, fruit suddenly tastes decadently sweet. Generally speaking 1–3 servings of fruit daily is fine. You don't want to binge on fruit because it *does* contain sugar, but since it also contains nutrition, there's no reason to avoid it either. The highest-quality fruit you can eat are berries. They contain more antioxidants than other fruit (and even some vegetables), and they contain less sugar than other fruit as well.

Do I have to buy organic fruits and vegetables? While organic is ideal, we all need to work within our budgets. When making shopping decisions, it helps to know which produce contains the least pesticide residue, and which contains the most. The Environmental Working Group (EWG) puts out a list every year of the Clean Fifteen and the Dirty Dozen. If you're going to buy conventional produce, choose from the Clean Fifteen. When it comes to the Dirty Dozen, it's best to choose organic. Why? Here's just one example: a single grape can contain 15 different types of pesticides, which is why it's on the list of conventional produce to avoid.

CLEAN FIFTEEN	DIRTY DOZEN
Asparagus	Apple
Avocado	Celery
Cabbage	Cucumber
Cantaloupe	Grape
Cauliflower	Nectarine
Grapefruit	Peach
Kiwi	Spinach
Mango	Strawberry
Onion	
Papaya	
Pineapple	
Sweet Potato	
* Eggplant, Peas and Corn are part of the Clean Fifteen, but they aren't allowed on the AIP.	* Bell Pepper, Cherry Tomatoes, Potatoes and Snap Peas are part of the dirty dozen, but we avoid them on the AIP anyway.

In our cookie-loving culture, you might be wondering, "Can I have cookies on the AIP?" Yes—in moderation. And I need to define moderation. That doesn't mean a few cookies every day. When you first start the AIP, try to find a balance between what you need to do to heal, and what you need to do to keep from feeling deprived. If having some AIP-friendly treats in the freezer keep you from reaching for junk food, then keep them stocked. Just don't binge on them. Just because they're gluten and dairy-free doesn't mean they're healing foods. They're treats, and eating too many will derail your healing. The good news is that most people find they crave dessert less and less, the longer they're on a healing diet. And many people make a major leap forward in their health when they remove them from their diet altogether.

That doesn't mean you don't get cake on your birthday. You do! And there are an amazing number of wonderful recipes available now, both online and in cookbooks. See the Resources chapter at the end of this book for details. You'll have many decadent choices available to you.

Coconut is the darling of the paleo AIP community, offering flour to bake with, oil to cook with, milk as a dairy alternative, aminos as a soy sauce substitute, and the meat itself as a recommended snack. In spite of its name, it's not a nut. However, some people have trouble if they eat too much. With the exception of the oil, it's recommended to consume in moderation: no more than 1 cup coconut milk daily, 1/4 cup coconut butter/coconut flakes daily, and 1/8 cup coconut flour daily.

Let's finish this chapter talking about nutrient-density, so it's foremost in your minds. The Standard American Diet (SAD) is made up of nutrient-poor foods: pasta, bread, hydrogenated oils, processed foods and junk food. The AIP is the opposite. Every bite we take is meant to contain nutrition that will help us heal. While everything allowed on the diet is healthy, some foods have special healing potential:

- **Seafood** contains high amounts of anti-inflammatory omega 3 fatty acids. Both Terry Wahls and Sarah Ballantyne recommend we eat approximately 1 lb. per week.

- **Organ meats** have 10–100 times the nutrition of other cuts of meat. It's a myth that they store toxins. Rather, they store the nutrition that our bodies need to *remove* toxins. Terry Wahls recommends we eat 12 oz. per week. Sarah Ballantyne recommends we make them a regular part of our diet, ideally eating them at least four times per week.

- **Bone broth** is traditionally made by simmering bones slowly for around 24 hours. This process pulls nutrition from the bones: marrow, collagen, gelatin, glycine, proline, hyaluronic acid, chondroitin sulfate, calcium, phosphorous, magnesium and potassium. They're building blocks for your body, and they're especially beneficial for reducing inflammation and helping our bodies heal. I have a recipe on my blog for the traditional method, as well as an Instant Pot method which pressure cooks the broth in just 2 hours: Phoenixhelix.com/recipes/.

- **Fermented foods** are rich in probiotics which help modulate the immune system, heal leaky gut, aid digestion, and act as anti-inflammatories. Eat some every day.

So, that's our healing diet in a nutshell, and the next page shows what it looks like in Food Pyramid form:

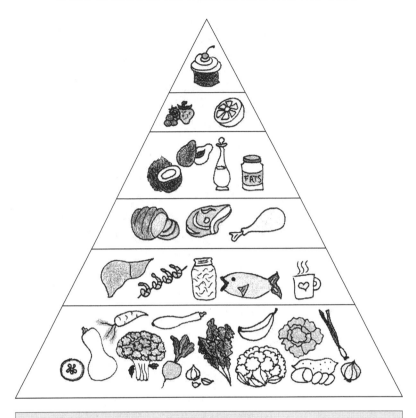

AIP FOOD PYRAMID

TOP: Desserts are reserved for special occasions

LEVEL 2: Fruit in moderation—1–3 servings

LEVEL 3: Healthy fats with every meal

LEVEL 4: Quality meats

LEVEL 5: Healing foods every day—organ meats, wild-caught seafood, fermented foods and bone broth

FOUNDATION: Vegetables—Eat 6–14 cups daily (measured raw)

CHAPTER 7

GROCERY LIST

Be sure to read the prior chapters that outline the foods to eat and the foods to avoid. You want to have a basic understanding of those categories so that you can make food decisions spontaneously, without referencing a list. The grocery list below is for your shopping convenience, but it's impossible to include every single food, especially when you take into account international markets. I've done my best!

PROTEIN		
Fish	Lamb	Duck
Shellfish	Pork	Pheasant
Beef	Chicken	Rabbit
Bison	Turkey	Venison

* Processed meats like bacon, sausage, jerky, hot dogs and deli meats, all usually contain nightshades in the form of paprika. Check ingredients carefully. We often have to source AIP-friendly versions online or make our own.

VEGETABLES	
Artichokes	Leeks
Arugula	Lettuce
Asparagus	Mushrooms
Avocado	Mustard Greens
Beets	Nopales
Bok Choy	Okra
Broccoli	Olives (pimento-free)
Broccolini	Onions
Brussels Sprouts	Parsnips
Cabbage	Plantains
Carrots	Pumpkin
Cauliflower	Radicchio
Celeriac	Radishes
Chard	Rapini
Chayote	Rhubarb
Collards	Rutabagas
Daikon Radish	Salsify
Endive	Scallions
Fennel	Spinach
Fiddleheads	Summer Squash
Garlic Scapes	Sunchokes
Jicama	Sweet Potatoes
Kale	Taro
Kohlrabi	Turnips

Watercress

Winter Squash

Yuca

Zucchini

FATS

Avocado Oil

Coconut Oil

Duck Fat

Extra-Virgin Olive Oil

Lard

Red Palm Oil

Schmaltz

Tallow

HERBS/SPICES

Basil

Bay Leaf

Chamomile

Chervil

Chives

Cilantro

Cinnamon

Cloves

Curry Leaf (not curry powder)

Dill Weed

Fenugreek

Garlic

Ginger

Horseradish

Kaffir Lime Leaf

Lavender

Lemon Balm

Lemongrass

Mace

Marjoram

Oregano

Onion Powder

Parsley

Peppermint

Rosemary

Saffron	Tarragon
Sage	Thyme
Savory	Truffle Salt
Sea Salt	Turmeric
Shallots	Vanilla (alcohol-free)
Spearmint	Wasabi

FRUIT (IN MODERATION)	
Apples	Guava
Apricots	Honeydew
Bananas	Huckleberries
Blackberries	Kiwi
Blueberries	Lemons
Cantaloupe	Limes
Cherries	Lychee
Coconut	Mango
Clementines	Nectarines
Cranberries	Oranges
Currants	Papaya
Dragonfruit	Peaches
Feijoa	Pears
Fresh Figs	Persimmons
Grapefruit	Pineapples
Grapes	Plums

Pomegranate	Star Fruit
Pomelo	Strawberries
Quince	Tangerines
Raspberries	Watermelon

BEVERAGES

Filtered Water	Honeybush Tea
Kombucha	Ginger Tea
Beet Kvass	Caffeinated Teas (in moderation): black, green, white, yerba mate
Water Kefir	
Rooibos Tea	

* Always check labels to be sure they're AIP-friendly.

SNACKS

Canned Seafood: salmon, tuna, sardines, oysters

Epic Bison Bacon Cranberry Bars

Wild Zora Lamb Rosemary Bars

Bacon's Heir Rosemary Pork Clouds

Sea Snax Original Flavor

Bare Fruit Cinnamon Apple Chips

Jacksons' Honest Sweet Potato Chips

Artisan Tropic Plantain Strips and Cassava Strips

PANTRY

Great Lakes Grass-Fed Gelatin and Collagen

Coconut Aminos

Red Boat Fish Sauce

Herbamare Seasoning Salt

Your Choice of Vinegars: apple cider, balsamic, champagne, coconut, red wine, sherry, ume plum, white wine

Aroy-D or Natural Value Coconut Milk and Coconut Cream (these are additive-free brands)

Coconut Butter

Dried Unsweetened Coconut

Sunfood Plain Coconut Wraps

AIP Flours: arrowroot, cassava, coconut, plantain, sweet potato, tapioca, tigernut

Other Baking Ingredients: carob powder and palm shortening

Natural Sweeteners: raw honey, pure maple syrup, molasses, dried fruit, date sugar, maple sugar, evaporated cane juice, sucanat

CHAPTER 8

THIS IS TOO HARD! I CAN'T DO IT!

It's common to have a moment of panic when you first read about the autoimmune protocol. I know I did! It's a lot of information, and it's a lot of restrictions. It's also natural to fear change, even when it's for the better. Thousands of people have done the AIP successfully, and you can too. Take a deep breath, and follow these five tips to make the transition easier:

1. **Focus on your goal.** You're trying to do what doctors say is impossible: reverse autoimmune disease. That's no small task. It makes sense that it's not easy to do. But it's certainly worthwhile. Look at your symptoms today. Is it worth doing this protocol if you can reduce them and possibly even make them go away altogether? Remember—nothing is harder than living with a disabling autoimmune disease. The AIP is a breeze by comparison.

2. **You can take it in phases.** We all have different personalities for making changes in our lives.

- **Some people are "all or nothing."** For them, diving right into the full AIP is the way to go.

- **Others (like me) find that too intimidating.** I started with a regular paleo diet (not the AIP), and you know what? Some people go into remission at that level. While that didn't happen for me, I did improve dramatically. My flares went from daily excruciating occurrences to moderate flares a few times per month. When I plateaued in my healing, I was ready for the added restrictions of the AIP, and I was rewarded for my efforts. My flares went away altogether. Do I wish I did the AIP sooner? No—I wasn't ready then. Taking it in phases was the right choice for me. You can do the same.

- **You are in charge of your healing journey.** If you're a rebel like me, it helps to remember that. No one is making you do this. It's totally your choice and your pace.

- **You can even take it in baby steps.** Remove one food category each week until you reach full AIP. Start with removing gluten, sugar and processed foods. Then remove grains and legumes. Then switch out refined oils for healthy fats. Next remove dairy. Then nightshades. Then eggs. Then alcohol. Then nuts and seeds (including coffee and cocoa). Finally remove the extra restrictions of *The Paleo Approach* (stevia, seed-based spices, etc.) You can also alter this order, choosing the easiest foods for you to give up first, and saving the hardest ones for last.

3. **Plan for it.** This is a big change, and it's not one you can easily do "on the fly." Decide when you'd like to begin. Finish reading this book before you start. And follow the steps in each chapter to make it easier. For example, you'll want to remove foods you can no longer eat and fill your kitchen with delicious healing foods before you even begin. You'll want to have plenty of AIP-friendly recipes to cook and an idea of what you'll eat for each meal during the week. Spontaneity and the AIP don't go well together.

4. **Get support.** While you are the only one who can make this change, it's a lot easier to do if the people you love support you. It's also helpful to find other people embarking on the AIP, who understand what you're going through. In Chapter 17, I give detailed advice for getting friends and family on board and also how to access the global AIP community.

5. **Nurture yourself.** Embarking on this kind of change can be stressful, so prioritize stress-relief and self-care. Some people believe they don't have time for this—they're too busy taking care of other people to take care of themselves. But here's the thing—if we don't take care of ourselves, we will become more and more disabled and unable to care for anyone else. There's a reason flight attendants tell us

to put our oxygen mask on first, before helping anyone else. It's a good symbol for healing. As I've mentioned in earlier chapters, stress can cause flares just as much as poor dietary choices. So, schedule time every week for something that brings you joy. And also take 15 minutes a day to yourself, every day, to do something relaxing. I give many suggestions for stress reduction in Chapter 20.

CHAPTER 9

AN AIP KITCHEN

Are you ready to get started? Let's tackle the kitchen first. It's about to become the most important room in your home.

- **Step 1: Remove the foods you can no longer eat.** This is the best scenario for succeeding on the AIP. Out of sight, out of mind really does work. I realize not everyone's family or roommates will agree to do this, but make the request. Your healing is worth it, and your friends and family can still eat whatever they want outside the house. They're just helping you by making your home AIP-friendly. If they don't agree, then it's time to do some negotiation. At the very least, ask that the kitchen be gluten-free, especially if you have celiac disease. The chance for gluten cross-contamination in a shared kitchen is extremely high, and that's a risk you don't want to take. After that, compartmentalize the kitchen. If most of your family is on-board and just one person isn't, maybe they can keep their foods in a special cabinet in the kitchen, one you will simply avoid. If the reverse is true, then store your food on certain shelves in the fridge, freezer and cabinets, so you don't have to reach past the takeout containers to get your ingredients for breakfast. Lastly, figure out which foods are the most tempting to you and ask that at least those foods be kept out of the house.

- **Step 2: Bring in the good stuff.** You want to fill your kitchen with the foods that support your healing. Use the grocery list in Chapter 7 as a guide.

- **Step 3: Become a label reader.** If you're anything like me, you believed that foods sold in the health food store were automatically healthy. I can't tell you how many times I fell for "vegetable source" listed on the ingredient list, as if that suddenly made an ingredient I couldn't pronounce safe to eat. In addition, health food store packages often contain gluten, soy, dairy, industrial oils and nightshades, among other things. Even herbal teas often contain soy lecithin. Isn't that crazy? On the AIP, you're going to be focusing more on whole foods and rarely buying foods in a package. Check the ingredients on everything you buy, and ideally don't buy any with more than one ingredient. Unnamed "spices" or "natural flavors" often include nightshades, and here's a list of common gluten ingredients to avoid: http://bit.ly/gluteningredients.

- **Step 4: Love your fridge and freezer.** There's a meme going around the internet that says, "Food with a shelf life isn't food." And a lot of the time, that's true. You are going to be buying mostly perishable foods because those are the foods your body is designed to eat. That means you will have a lot of empty space in your cupboards, and your fridge and freezer are going to be packed full. If you can afford a chest freezer, that's a great way to buy things in bulk when they're on sale and freeze leftovers from batch cooking sessions.

- **Step 5: Handy AIP kitchen tools.** You don't need fancy kitchen equipment to follow this diet. One of my friends writes the blog Slightly Lost Girl, and she followed this diet from a tiny kitchen in Mexico for two years, with just one knife and a few well-used pots and pans. But if you can afford it (or find it on Craigslist), there are some tools that can make your life a little easier:

  - **Mason jars with plastic reusable caps:** I think these are my favorite kitchen items. I store everything in them: fermented foods, bone broth, mason jar salads, leftovers. If you buy the wide-mouth jars, they're even freezer safe if you leave a couple of inches free at the top of the jar and don't put the caps on until they've frozen.

  - **Some sharp knives:** You're going to be cutting a lot of fresh meats and vegetables. Make it easy on yourself.

  - **Food processor:** This magic tool can make every-thing from cauliflower "rice" to liver paté to vegetable chips. It's like having your own little sous chef in the kitchen.

- **Immersion blender:** Most people don't like drinking bone broth straight-up, which means lots of delicious soups. An immersion blender is an easy way to purée creamy soups and gravies, right in the pan.

- **Spiralizer:** This kitchen tool isn't necessary, but it's definitely fun, and if you have a family, kids love spiralized vegetables. It's a great way to get them to eat more veggies, and it makes giving up pasta easy.

- **Instant pot:** This is the top wish list item for most people following the AIP. It's a lot of kitchen appliances in one: a slow cooker, pressure cooker, yogurt maker, vegetable steamer, and more. The slow cooker feature lets you start a meal when you leave for work and have it waiting for you when you get home at dinnertime. The pressure cooker is a huge time saver, letting you cook roasts in just 90 minutes and bone broth in just 2 hours.

- **My blog's Healing Store:** If you can't find these kitchen tools locally, I provide links to companies who sell them online: Phoenixhelix.com/store.

CHAPTER 10

FINDING NEW FLAVORS: AIP SPICES, HERBS AND SAUCES

One of the toughest transitions to the paleo autoimmune protocol is losing your favorite sauces and spices. When you start clearing out your kitchen and reading labels, soy sauce is the first thing to go, and most dressings, condiments and store-bought sauces follow. Next you look in your spice cabinet and sadly set aside the nightshades first: cayenne, chili powder, paprika, red pepper, store-bought curry and many other store-bought spice blends. Fruit-based and seed-based spices go next: allspice, anise seed, star anise, annatto, caraway, cardamom, celery seed, coriander, cumin, fennel seed, fenugreek, juniper, mustard, nutmeg, pepper (black, white, green and pink), poppy seeds, sesame seeds and vanilla bean.

As you stare forlornly into your cabinets, a common mistake is to just "make do" with no added flavors, and before you know it, you're eating bland food, resenting this diet, and feeling like the fun has been sucked out of your kitchen. Don't do that!

Let me reassure you: AIP food can be absolutely delicious and full of flavor. You just need to re-stock your cabinets with things you can eat, and experiment with new flavor profiles until you find new favorites.

First, look at the grocery list in Chapter 7. There are 37 herbs and spices allowed on the AIP. That's a lot! Start buying a few each week and incorporating them into your meals. If you have a health food store nearby, they usually sell herbs and spices in bulk very cheaply. You can buy a little at a time, often for less than a dollar. If you have room for an herb garden, get planting. And don't be afraid to use a LOT of herbs, especially when they're fresh. There's also an AIP-friendly seasoning salt called Herbamare that you can find in most health food stores.

Are you a cook who loves spicy heat in recipes—food with a kick? Without nightshades and peppercorns, you might wonder how to achieve that. Get familiar with these 4 AIP-friendly flavors:

1. **Fresh Ginger:** This is one of my favorites, and if you add a lot to a dish, it adds a nice amount of heat. The key is to grate it very finely with a ceramic grater (which releases a lot of hot ginger juice). Or put the ginger in your freezer and use a microplane to zest it. An added bonus is that ginger is anti-inflammatory.

2. **Horseradish:** This is one of my husband's favorite flavors. Store-bought brands, unfortunately, contain additives. However, it's pretty easy to make your own in a food processor. Buy some fresh horseradish root, peel it and

cut into cubes. Add to the food processor with just 1–2 tablespoons of water until it turns into a paste. This crushing action starts an enzyme activity that releases "hot" oils from the horseradish. Vinegar halts this process. If you like your horseradish mild, add 1 Tbsp. white wine vinegar and a pinch of sea salt right away; pulse to blend. If you like your horseradish hot, let it sit for 10 minutes before adding the vinegar and salt. Transfer to a jar and refrigerate. It should keep well for about 4 weeks.

3. **Wasabi:** This is another AIP-friendly hot condiment. If you can find it fresh, you grate it similarly to ginger, but be aware that it loses its heat in about 20 minutes. You can also buy it freeze-dried with this additive-free brand: Sushi Sonic.

4. **Garlic:** The finer you mince garlic, the more intense the heat, especially if you smash the clove first. Using a garlic press releases the most flavor. Bonus tip: If you heat garlic immediately after mincing, it still tastes good but loses most of its medicinal property. However, if you mince your garlic and wait 10 minutes before cooking, it has a chance to release plenty of allicin (the healing compound), and once released it's not destroyed by heat. Garlic cooks fast though, so watch it closely. Burnt garlic tastes bitter.

Next up: sauces. Coconut Aminos and Red Boat Fish Sauce are your friends. The aminos add a sweet-savory flavor to a dish, and the fish sauce adds a salty-savory flavor. You can use them separately or together. A 1:1 blend is a great soy sauce substitute.

Have fun with vinegar: Most of us are used to the basic vinegars (balsamic, wine and apple cider), and they're wonderful! But there's a world of vinegar out there, and each one imparts its own flavor. The only ones to avoid are the grain-based ones (like rice, malt and distilled white vinegar). I can recommend three AIP-friendly ones to try: coconut, sherry and ume plum. A note on the ume plum: it's sweet, salty and sour at the same time. When you experiment with it, start with small quantities and remove the salt from your recipe. Soon, you might have a new favorite.

Lastly, in the resource section of this book, I'll be sharing online AIP recipe resources as well as top-notch AIP cookbooks. People have walked this path before you, and they are people who LOVE food. They've learned how to maximize the flavors on this diet and will show you how to do the same. **And if you visit the recipes page on my blog, you'll find a recipe roundup of 50 AIP-friendly condiment recipes:** Phoenixhelix.com/recipes. You don't have to live without ketchup, mayonnaise, salsa, or any of your favorite flavor boosts. You just need to learn new ways to make them.

CHAPTER 11

WHAT WILL I EAT? SAMPLE MENUS

EXAMPLE 1	
Breakfast	**Skillet Breakfast** Made with leftover meat and vegetables from last night's dinner, and a cup of bone broth on the side
Lunch	**Large Salad** With greens, vegetables, avocado, canned salmon and olive oil vinaigrette
Dinner	**Roast Chicken and Root Vegetables** With a cup of beet kvass on the side
Snack (if needed)	**Fresh Berries with Coconut Whipped Cream**

EXAMPLE 2	
Breakfast	**Homemade Chicken and Vegetable Soup** Prepared in a big batch to last all week
Lunch	**Herbed Beef Patty** On a portabello bun with bacon and guacamole; sweet potato chips on the side
Dinner	**Shrimp Curry** Made with homemade curry blend, served over cauliflower-rice, with a glass of kombucha on the side
Snack (if needed)	**Kale Chips and Sardines**

EXAMPLE 3	
Breakfast	**Plantain Pancakes** And a small collagen green smoothie
Lunch	**Chicken Liver Paté** With raw vegetables for dipping

Dinner	**Slow Cooker Roast Pork** With onion-apple gravy, sautéed asparagus, and some sauerkraut on the side
Snack (if needed)	**Epic Bison Bacon Cranberry Bar and Original Sea Snax**

As you can see from those examples, your menu on the AIP can be wide-ranging and delicious. Let me touch on some key elements in my examples that I'd like you to notice:

- **Breakfasts:** This is the meal that leaves most newbies wondering what to eat. When you can't have eggs or grains (and therefore no cereal, waffles or oatmeal), what's left? I showed you three different examples above. Leftovers are the quickest and easiest breakfast. Soup's my personal favorite, and while it may seem strange to you, many cultures start their day with soup. It's nourishing, nurturing and satiating at the same time. As for missing grains, you actually can have cereal, waffles and "oatmeal" on the AIP—or at least grain-free versions of them. There's an e-cookbook called 85 Amazing AIP Breakfasts: http://bit.ly/aipbreakfasts. It contains recipes for hot cereals, cold cereal, pancakes, waffles, cinnamon rolls, herbal "coffee," smoothies, plus a wide variety of meat patties, skillet meals and delicious soups. If you do decide to go with pancakes or cereal, just be sure you balance your breakfast with some protein. You'll notice in my example above, I added a collagen smoothie, but a couple of meat patties on the side works too.

- **Batch Cooking/Leftovers:** On the AIP, you're going to be cooking most (if not all) of your meals. That requires a lot more time in the kitchen, and you want to be as efficient as possible. This is where batch cooking comes in handy. Always make extra. If you're roasting vegetables, roast two trays instead of one. If you're making burger patties or sausage patties, prepare 2–3 pounds at a time; you can freeze them uncooked, and then pop them in a skillet for a quick meal. Make big pots of soup and enjoy it all week. Roast a couple of chickens at a time, shred the meat, and eat it with different vegetables and toppings for a quick breakfast or lunch. And when it comes to fresh vegetables, chop them in advance. If you set aside a few hours on weekends to prep and cook, you'll have everything you need for quick meals on weekdays. If you're new to batch cooking and want more guidance, AIP Batch Cook is an online video tutorial, which includes recipes and meal plans: http://bit.ly/batchcooking.

- **Slow Cookers and Pressure Cookers:** I mentioned these in the AIP Kitchen chapter, but they're worth mentioning again because they make life so much easier. A slow cooker is like having a personal chef. You add your ingredients in the morning, go to work, and when you come home, dinner's ready. Pressure cookers are all about speed. You can make 24-hour bone broth in just 2 hours, cook a roast in 90 minutes, and cook vegetables in just a few minutes. An Instant Pot is both a slow cooker and a pressure cooker in one. You can find links to both of these in my blog store: Phoenixhelix.com/store.

- **AIP Food Pyramid (Nutrient Density):** If you look at my menus, you'll see I followed the food pyramid from Chapter 6. There are vegetables at every meal, and by the end of the day, you want to have eaten a wide variety. You'll also see that I incorporated healing foods daily: bone broth, organ meat, wild-caught seafood, and fermented foods and beverages. Macronutrients are also important: every meal and snack includes some healthy fat and protein. This is because balanced blood sugar is essential to healing. What we eat is just as important as what we don't.

- **A Little Convenience:** We are lucky to have some AIP-friendly store-bought snacks available now. The Epic Bison Bacon Cranberry Bar in the third sample menu is a pemmican protein bar that is "Paleo Approach Approved." And Sea Snax Original are AIP-friendly seaweed chips. You can find these and others in my blog store as well. When you cook as much as we do, any convenience is a gift: Phoenixhelix.com/store.

- **Balancing the Old with the New:** Any time you make a change this big, there's a learning curve. After you've been on the AIP a little while, you'll find favorite recipes and get into a cooking groove that doesn't require so much planning. Just be sure you don't get into a food rut. The more variety we eat, the better our nutrition because every single food has a unique nutritional profile. I host a weekly AIP recipe roundtable on my blog, Phoenixhelix.com, where we share a combination of creative and simple meals. The goal is to inspire each other to try something new at least once a week.

- **Meal Plans:** The samples above give you an idea of what a daily menu can look like. Personally, I sit down once a week and write out my meal plan for 7 days: all 3 meals plus snacks. Then, I write up my grocery list from the plan, and I'm never caught with an empty fridge, wondering what to eat. If you're new to meal planning, or you have brain fog and can't manage it right now, there are monthly AIP meal plans you can buy. You can find them in my blog store as well: Phoenixhelix.com/store.

CHAPTER 12

FREQUENTLY ASKED QUESTIONS

Why can't I just take an allergy test?

I wish we could just take a test—that would be so much easier! The autoimmune protocol addresses food intolerances, which are different from allergies. Food allergies can be life-threatening, sending people to the hospital in anaphylactic shock, and it is possible to test for those. Intolerances, on the other hand, ramp up inflammation in the body over time, exacerbating the symptoms of autoimmune disease. Unfortunately, there is no scientifically proven lab test for food intolerances. Although there are tests sold under the names IgG, Alcat, Enterolab, EAV and Muscle Testing, these tests often give both false positives and false negatives. For that reason, an elimination diet (like the AIP) is the gold standard for discovering food intolerances. It takes effort, but it's your only guarantee of accurate results.

Is the AIP Forever? Do I have to eat this way for life?

No. The AIP is an elimination diet with two phases: elimination and reintroduction. During the reintroduction phase, you learn which foods your body does and doesn't tolerate. I'll go over this process in detail in Chapter 24. Some foods you'll be able to welcome back into your diet on a daily basis. Some foods you'll be able to eat occasionally. And some foods you'll learn you need to avoid altogether. However, as we heal, we are often able to tolerate a wider variety of foods. That means if a food reintroduction fails the first time around, it might be successful 6 or 12 months later. The goal is always to expand our diet safely; the more diverse our food, the more diverse our nutrition. We just don't want to eat foods that cause our autoimmune symptoms to worsen.

With that in mind, there are some foods you will want to avoid forever. Gluten is one of them. The same goes for processed foods and fake ingredients. You won't be returning to a junk food-laden SAD diet. Instead, most people will settle on a paleo-style diet, personalized for them.

How soon will I see results?

It varies. Some people notice improvement immediately. For others it takes a few months. There are 4 things you can do to maximize the healing impact of this diet: (1) Do it 100%—no cheating. The AIP doesn't work as a part-time protocol. (2) Don't just avoid foods. Put thought into the foods you *do* eat. We can't heal without nutrition, so choosing nutrient-dense foods speeds the healing process. (3) Address lifestyle factors as well as diet. They are just as important when it comes to reversing autoimmune disease, and I'll be sharing tips for those in later chapters. (4) Keep a symptom journal. Often we only notice what's still wrong, and we miss what's gotten better. Writing down a summary of how you're feeling, and seeing how that changes month to month, helps you see and celebrate your progress. I give you details on what to include in your journal in Chapter 23.

If after three months, you still haven't seen improvement, it's time to do some troubleshooting. I share troubleshooting tips in Chapter 26.

Do I really need to eat organ meat?

While the quickest path to healing is nutrient-dense AIP, you are in charge of your healing journey. You don't have to implement everything at once, and if you find organ meat intimidating, you can postpone that for a little while. Just remember that nutrition is key to healing, and organ meats are 10–100 times more nutritious than other cuts of meat. If you're not ready to eat them yet, start including other healing foods instead: wild-caught seafood, fermented foods, bone broth, and a wide variety of vegetables.

When you're ready to try organ meat, I recommend starting with chicken livers. They're a mild flavor, cook quickly, and are relatively easy to find.

Can I stop my medications when I start this diet?

The short answer is no. Healing through diet and lifestyle takes time, and if you go off your medication before your body has a chance to heal, you will most likely have an autoimmune flare. The one exception might be people who start the AIP immediately after diagnosis, before going on medication. Sometimes it's possible to avoid meds at this stage, but not always. Work closely with your doctor when making this decision.

That said, the goal for many of us is to reduce or eliminate our need for medication. So, how long does this take? It varies. Your symptoms need to go away before your medication does. Dr. Terry Wahls says that blood pressure and blood sugar medications are often the first prescriptions that can be reduced. Autoimmune medication takes longer. Autoimmune disease usually builds in the body for years before diagnosis. It makes sense that it will take time to reverse this process. Wait until your symptoms improve before approaching your doctor about potentially reducing your medication.

Steroids are meant to be taken short-term to control autoimmune flares, and they're a good first choice to try eliminating once your flares have stopped. However, you'll want to slowly taper your dose under a doctor's supervision, to minimize any rebound effect. DMARDs are designed to be taken long-term and many are often prescribed simultaneously. Some people have been able to get off DMARDs altogether, while others have been able to reduce their numbers and dosage over time.

If you have Hashimoto's or Addison's disease, you might need to stay on your medication. We need the hormones from our thyroid and adrenal glands to function, and when those glands are damaged, they stop producing enough. Some people are diagnosed before much damage is done, and they are able to remain (or become) medication-free. Others are diagnosed after many years of damage, and therefore medication is needed long-term. If that is you, the key is finding the right brand and dose that works best for you.

Please know that there is no shame in taking medication. Autoimmune disease is serious business, and while the side effects of medication can be scary, living with the symptoms of an untreated autoimmune disease is even scarier. There's a wise saying: Seek progress, not perfection. Sometimes success on the AIP is eliminating medication. Other times, it's a combination of diet and medication, where diet eliminates the symptoms that medication alone couldn't address. Both types of success are cause for celebration. No matter what, never change your medications without consulting your physician.

If I have a flare, does that mean the AIP isn't working for me?

This bears repeating: healing takes time. And it's actually quite normal to continue to flare when you first start the AIP. Flares are a result of an overactive immune system, and it takes time to calm the immune system down. Look for your flares to reduce in number and intensity. For me, I started with daily excruciating flares. Slowly, they reduced to a few times per week and eventually a few times per month. At the same time, they reduced from excruciating to moderate to mild. However, it was a full year before they went away altogether. If you see no improvement in your flares after three months, read the troubleshooting tips in Chapter 26.

Where do supplements fit on the AIP?

Supplements are complicated. We're used to thinking of them as supportive of health, but that's not always the case. Follow these simple rules while on the AIP:

1. Read labels carefully. Many supplements contain gluten, soy, dairy and other ingredients not allowed on the AIP. While you may have removed these foods from your diet, you might be unknowingly consuming them in supplement form. Look for allergy statements on the bottle, and if you don't recognize an ingredient, look it up to determine its source.

2. When it comes to vitamins and minerals, seek to get these through food rather than supplements. Nutrition is designed to work in synergy. Plants and proteins are a complex blend of nutrients that work together to provide our bodies with the building blocks for health. Isolating one of those into supplement form and taking it separately can throw our bodies out of balance. The one exception is magnesium, which is difficult to get through diet alone.

3. Here are the categories where supplements might help people with autoimmune disease: digestive support, pain relief, immune system regulation, and support of any organs affected by your disease. Work with a healthcare practitioner to help you choose the best supplement for you. Examine.com is also a great online resource that offers free, unbiased research into supplement effectiveness.

4. Always introduce just one supplement at a time. While the goal is for supplements to help us, sometimes they harm us, and even more frequently they have no effect whatsoever. If you introduce a bunch at once and have a negative reaction, you won't know what's causing it. The same is true if you have a positive response—you might end up taking a number of supplements that do nothing, because you can't identify the one that's helpful.

5. Don't take too many supplements. Some naturopaths are supplement-crazy, and they send people home with grocery sacks full of pills. Just because they are "natural" doesn't mean they're harmless. Most of us with autoimmune disease have compromised digestion and compromised detoxification pathways. That means it's very difficult for our bodies to process high quantities of pills in any form. So, choose wisely the few supplements that work best for you.

6. Supplement needs change over time. Just because you need a supplement now, doesn't mean you'll need it forever. As your body heals and your digestion improves, and your autoimmune disease reverses, your supplement needs will change accordingly.

Can I do the AIP as a vegetarian?

The short answer is no. Protein is a necessary food group, and the AIP eliminates most vegetarian protein sources (grains, soy, eggs, legumes, dairy, nuts and seeds). These are eliminated because they commonly irritate digestion and/or trigger autoimmune symptoms. Also, the AIP is a diet that focuses on nutrient-density, and both meat and seafood contain vital nutrients that are more bioavailable than those same nutrients found in plants (such as iron, zinc and vitamins A, B12 and D). Similarly, the omega 3 fatty acids found in seafood are much more bioavailable than those found in plants. Many long-term vegetarians end up being deficient in those nutrients, and they are all essential to healing.

If you're finding the transition to eating meat difficult, know that you're not alone. Many people have walked this path before you. Terry Wahls was a vegetarian for 20 years before turning to paleo for her health. Many of my AIP blogging friends were vegan. All of them felt dramatically better after reintroducing meat and/or seafood into their diet.

That said, I know it's not easy. Here are some tips to help you through the transition:

- Seafood is one of the easiest proteins to digest, so it's a good first choice. You can follow the AIP as a pescatarian and continue to avoid meat.
- If you were a vegetarian for ethical reasons, you might be interested in *The Vegetarian Myth*, a book which talks about ethics from the opposite perspective. You can also make ethical choices about the meat you do eat, choosing meat from animals that were humanely raised. Get to

know your local farmers and their farming practices, and shop from the best.

- Many long-term vegans and vegetarians have depleted stomach acid, and we need stomach acid to digest our food completely. You can increase your stomach acid naturally by taking a tablespoon of apple cider vinegar in a small amount of water before and/or after your meals. If that's not enough, work with a nutritionist on HCL supplementation.

- When it comes to meat, start with homemade meat stock or bone broth. When you're comfortable with that, make a soup with meat and vegetables and blend it all together into a thick soup. When you're comfortable with that, don't blend it—eat the meat and vegetables in chunks. When you're comfortable with that, move onto stews and slow-braised meats (like roasts in the slow cooker). Meat cooked slowly at low temperatures, in broth or natural juices, is easier to digest than fried or grilled meats. Those would be the last ones to reintroduce.

- You may find that you're able to make the transition quickly, or it may take you many months of baby steps to become comfortable with this new style of eating. Keep your health your focus, and take whatever time you need.

If I fall off the AIP wagon, do I have to start over on day one?

Unfortunately, yes. I'm sorry. I don't say this to be mean. The science of an elimination diet is that you need to avoid the foods for a minimum of 30 consecutive days. This is the only way your immune system has a chance to calm down enough to communicate tolerance and intolerance clearly during reintroductions. If you fall off the wagon, just get right back on. Many people take a few tries before getting solidly on the protocol. When you're ready, you'll be able to do it.

If you really struggle with this, read Chapter 16: Overcoming Self-Sabotage. There's also an online group coaching program called SAD to AIP in SIX. It provides guidance and support for the transition to AIP, and many people succeed in that group, who previously failed on their own: http://bit.ly/aipclass.

CHAPTER 13

EATING AT RESTAURANTS

For the first 30 days, avoid eating outside your home if possible. The only way you can know 100% what you're eating is if you are the one preparing your food. At a restaurant, there are a number of variables: a wide variety of staff members involved in the preparation of your food and a wide variety of ingredients. It's easy for mistakes to be made, even when your requests are clear. While I will share tips for making the safest choices possible in a restaurant, the AIP is an elimination diet. The only way to know if it's working for you is if you are sure you are avoiding all of the restricted foods.

Once you've become comfortable with the AIP and have started feeling some improvements, you can experiment with restaurants. They shouldn't be a regular part of your routine, but it's nice to have an option for dining out occasionally. Depending on where you live, you might actually have a paleo restaurant option. They are becoming more common in some of the larger cities like Berkeley (Mission Heirloom), Portland (Cultured Caveman), Austin (Picnik), Berlin (Sauvage), and Sydney (Paleo Café), to name a few. Google is your friend. Search paleo + your hometown and see what turns up.

If there is no paleo restaurant available and let's face it—that's true for most of us—what do you do?

- **Step 1:** Choose a restaurant that focuses on fresh, local ingredients if possible. Not only are you supporting your local farmers, but these are people who care about food, are more likely to be educated about food allergies, and will accommodate accordingly. Eatwellguide.org is a great website for locating these restaurants.

- **Step 2:** Ask for the gluten-free menu. Gluten is in a surprising number of spices, sauces and dressings. This will make your menu decisions much easier.

- **Step 3:** Respect your waiter. Before you order, tell them you're a high-maintenance customer but you tip well (and be sure you do). Use the "allergy" word because they take that seriously. Restaurant staff are busy people, so make your questions as simple as possible. Don't explain autoimmune disease or the AIP or every single item you can't have. Instead, look at the menu, choose something that looks like it fits the protocol, and then ask them a few questions to clarify.

- **Step 4:** So what are some good AIP choices? (1) Salad—order extra meat and olive oil/vinegar dressing, and ask them to skip the tomatoes and peppers. (2) Plain bunless burger with avocado on the side. (3) Grilled meat or seafood with extra veggies on the side. (4) Avoid all menu selections with breading or sauces. (5) When you place your order, say you are allergic to gluten, soy, dairy and red pepper spices. Ask them to check with the chef to see if your menu selection includes any of these things. They might need to adjust their seasonings or skip seasoning altogether. It's always helpful to bring some AIP-friendly flavoring with you, like Herbamare seasoned salt. Lastly, many restaurants use butter in a lot of their cooking, so ask them to use olive oil instead. If you've been able to reintroduce some foods (see Chapter 24), your menu choices might become more varied.

As you can see, it's not easy to eat AIP in restaurants. But many people who have been at this a long time say that they eventually find a restaurant locally where the owners and staff get to know them, and they can trust they will be served food safely. That's the goal for us all.

CHAPTER 14
TRAVELING ON THE AIP

Once you get into a groove with the autoimmune protocol, your kitchen becomes your happy place. It's where you can always find safe and delicious food.

Then come travel plans, and our safe kitchens are left behind. "Paleo road food" is an oxymoron, so how do we manage to eat well away from home? If you don't have autoimmune disease, you can lighten up when you travel, do the best you can, and get back on track when you return. But when eating the wrong food can bring on an autoimmune flare, what are you supposed to do? First, don't let fear stop you from traveling. Whether it's a business trip, a visit to family, or a vacation you've been dreaming about for years, you can do this! You just need a plan.

STEP 1: GETTING THERE

- **Traveling By Car:** The best thing about road travel is that you have more room to bring food with you. A cooler is your friend. If you're only driving one or two days to get to your destination, it's possible to bring along all the food you need. Here are some ideas:

- Fermented foods like sauerkraut and kombucha in mason jars.
- Precooked burger patties and chicken.
- Canned tuna, sardines, or oysters. Don't forget the can opener! You can also buy pouched tuna and salmon from Vital Choice Seafood and skip the can opener.
- AIP frozen meals from Paleo on the Go.
- AIP protein bars: (1) Epic Bacon Bison Cranberry Bar (2) Wild Zora Lamb Rosemary Bar or (3) Plain Jerky from US Wellness Meats.
- Precut raw vegetables and fruit.
- Coconut flakes and dried fruit.
- Mason jar salads, extra virgin olive oil, and your favorite vinegar.
- Gelatin gummy candies and some AIP baked treats, to ward off the temptation of roadside indulgences.
- Some AIP crunchy snacks: (1) Bacon's Heir Rosemary Pork Clouds, (2) Artisan Tropic Cinnamon Plantain Strips, or (3) Jackson's Honest Sweet Potato Chips.
- Sea salt and your favorite AIP-friendly spices.
- Water bottles, travel mugs, and your favorite gluten-free teas.
- Be sure and bring some plates and silverware as well. And if you have room for a slow cooker, that can make cooking easy once you reach your destination.
- My blog's Healing Store includes links to the

convenience foods and vendors listed above:
Phoenixhelix.com/store.

- **Traveling By Plane:** For short trips, one packed meal is enough to get you to your destination. For long trips, it might be several. Prioritize space in your carry-on bags for food, and include a small reusable ice pack to keep your food fresh. Alternately, you can also freeze your food so it doubles as an ice pack and eat it as it defrosts. Eat the fresh food at the beginning of your trip, and save shelf-stable food like jerky or canned fish for later in the trip. Look at the list above for meal ideas.

STEP 2: LODGING

- **Full Kitchen:** If you can find and afford lodging with a full kitchen this is ideal. Vrbo.com lists vacation rental property (houses and condos), all of which should have a full kitchen. Airbnb.com lists rooms for rent in people's homes, some of which are separate entrance apartments and guesthouses with full kitchens. There are hotel chains where every room has a full kitchen, such as Residence Inn and Homewood Suites. And there's also a group on Facebook of people around the world who follow the AIP, who are willing to host guests who are traveling: Facebook.com/groups/PaleoAIPhosting.

- **Kitchenette:** If a full kitchen's not an option, seek lodging with a microwave and mini-fridge. Most hotel/motel chains have at least a few rooms with this option, and some chains offer this in every room, like Embassy Suites. You can bring a slow cooker or Instant Pot along, and expand your cooking options even more.

- **Hotel:** If you find yourself stuck in a hotel without even a kitchenette, choose a restaurant nearby (or onsite) where you can speak to the manager and chef about eating safely during your stay. Follow the restaurant advice in the previous chapter.

- **With Friends or Family:** If you're staying at someone's home, you automatically have access to a kitchen, which is great! The challenge here is meeting your own dietary needs surrounded by people who likely aren't paleo. Here are my tips:

  - Keep the diet conversation as simple as possible. Tell them that you're on a special diet for health reasons and that certain foods increase your autoimmune symptoms. For that reason, you can't eat the same food they do.

  - Don't expect them to adapt their diet for you. Instead, plan on preparing your own meals. Just ask for some room in the fridge, tell them you'll cook something simple for yourself, and then share their table and enjoy their company at mealtimes.

  - At this point, your host might offer to adapt their meals to include you. If this happens, come up with some simple meal ideas everyone can enjoy. (Almost everyone loves meat and vegetables.) Be sure to help with the cooking, both to share the work, and to ensure no inflammatory ingredients accidentally slip into the meal. Don't be disappointed if your host doesn't offer, however. Some people find it too intimidating to meet the needs of a special diet. Thankfully, you can take care of yourself.

○ Be careful to avoid cross-contamination. Use separate pans and cutting boards to prepare your food, and avoid things like grills that may contain gluten residue.

○ One drawback of staying with friends and family is that you might be surrounded by SAD foods that you're tempted to eat, even though they hurt you. In those moments, get up and go for a walk or do an activity outside of the house. If you know in advance the temptation will be overwhelming, choose to stay at a hotel or vacation rental instead.

STEP 3: SOURCING FOOD

● **Eat Well Guide:** This website is a great travel resource. It has listings for health food stores, farmers markets and restaurants who use quality ingredients. Just type in the zip code of your travel destination to see what options await your arrival: Eatwellguide.org.

- **Grocery Stores:** Whole Foods is a haven for paleo travelers. With over 370 locations across the country, there will often be one near your travel destination. Search the store locator on their website. In addition to quality meat, seafood, fruits and vegetables, they have some AIP prepared foods for a quick meal: (1) Build-your-own salad bar (2) Rotisserie chickens and deli meats—choose from their Naked line to avoid nightshade spices. If there's no Whole Foods where you're going, no worries. Just find the best grocery store you can and shop the perimeter for fresh food offerings.

- **Markets:** Grocery stores aren't your only option. Farmers markets are common across the country now. Ethnic markets are a great place to find inexpensive food and some paleo favorites like plantains. If you're on the coast, fresh fish markets can't be beat.

- **Restaurants:** See the previous chapter for tips.

STEP 4: MINDBODY

- **Let Go of Perfectionism:** You're not at home, so you can't control your food completely. Accept this, and prioritize what's most important to you. I don't worry about eating organically when I travel. Refined oils don't make me flare, so I don't worry about those either. But gluten, dairy and nightshades can put me in a lot of pain very quickly, so I'm very careful about those. The more you get to know your own body, the more you'll be able to make your own personalized priorities.

- **Protect Your Sleep:** One of the biggest factors in autoimmune healing is how well (and how much) we sleep. Travel is hard on sleep: different beds, different time zones, lots of new activities. Our bodies like routine, so this can throw our sleep out of whack. However, there are steps we can take to sleep as well as possible:
  - Prioritize sleep in your travel plans. You may have been someone who took red-eye flights in the past, or got up at pre-dawn to hit the road for a long day of travel. Now your body has different needs. Avoid travel too early or too late in the day, if possible.
  - Bring some things with you that can help you sleep better: a familiar pillow, a white noise machine, an eye mask, ear plugs, and an herbal tea like passionflower that's relaxing, to sip at night.
- **Master the Art of Relaxation:** Vacations are meant to be fun! Prepare the best you can, and then just let go and have a good time. The more you relax, the better you will feel. It's scientific truth that relaxation turns off inflammatory genes. Soak it in!

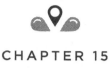

CHAPTER 15

AIP HOLIDAYS

The holidays are meant to be about beautiful things: celebration, love, family, fellowship. But they come wrapped in a package that includes stress, pressure and a tradition of foods we can no longer eat. So, how does an AIP Warrior survive? We plan for the temptations and stresses, and go out of our way to boost our reserves and stay flare-free this season.

Temptation #1 Holiday Treats: Most of us have very specific foods we associate with the holidays, and we crave them. It might be Christmas cookies and candy canes, potato latkes and doughnuts, collard greens and black-eyed peas, or sheer khurma and Turkish delight. While we can't eat the traditional versions of these recipes, we can find or create AIP versions to enjoy. In the AIP food pyramid, dessert is at the top because it's meant to make up only a small part of our diet—special occasions as opposed to every day. Well, the holidays are the perfect time of year to enjoy them. We're much less likely to binge on the foods that will really hurt us, if we allow ourselves some holiday treats that won't. The good news is that there are literally thousands of AIP recipes available now—both online and in cookbooks. Whatever food you're craving, someone else is craving it too. Google is your friend: type in AIP and the name of the recipe, and you will likely find what you seek. I also have a dessert Pinterest board which you can find here: Pinterest.com/eileen1365. Treat yourself for the holidays, just don't binge. Remember, just because it's made from natural sugars doesn't make it a health food.

Temptation #2 Holiday Meals: So that's the treats, but what about the meals themselves, filled with foods you no longer eat? You have options:

1. You can offer to host and cook the meal. This is the safest choice food-wise, but the toughest one time and energy-wise. Only do this if you feel you have plenty of both.

2. Depending on your family or friends, they might be willing to make the holiday meal AIP. You can work together on meal planning, grocery shopping, and cooking on the big day. It's a way people can show their love and support for you, and you all share the effort. You can even ask that to be your gift for the holiday.

3. Bring your own food with you. This is the simplest solution. You only need to prepare food for yourself. No one else has to change their plans. You just heat up your food when you arrive, and enjoy their company at the table. However, if you're going to be miserable seeing a table full of foods you can't eat, this isn't the choice for you.

4. If a restaurant or catering company is involved, communicate your needs by either choosing the place, the

menu or speaking with the chef to request a special meal for you.

5. Lastly, we get lots of invitations over the holiday season; it's okay to decline the ones that are more stressful than fun.

Temptation #3 Alcohol: Look ahead at your social calendar. Where will alcohol be served? For those situations, bring your own delicious and safe beverage with you. It might be kombucha, holiday cider, fruit-infused water, or anything else you enjoy. Bringing your own drink serves two purposes: it keeps you from feeling deprived, and it prevents others from asking you why you're not drinking. Generally speaking, as long as your glass is full, people don't notice whether it's alcoholic or not.

Stress #1 Time: We don't have enough of it, right? It's a universal feeling that intensifies over the holiday season. Here's the thing: the length of our day isn't going to change, so the way to manage this stress is to learn to say no and limit the amount of extra tasks you take on. Sometimes this feels beyond your control, but it's not. Saying no gets easier with practice, and if you have trouble prioritizing, enlist the help of an objective friend.

Stress #2 Money: Although the holiday season started as a spiritual celebration, it's become the season of gift-giving, and we often put pressure on ourselves to give extravagantly. This can lead to a second job or high debt, both of which can be autoimmune flare triggers. It takes more thought and creativity to give someone a gift they will love that doesn't cost a lot of money, but it's absolutely possible. Start brainstorming now for ideas. It's also okay to set new expectations.

If you have kids, let them know the budget is tighter and ask them to choose 1 or 2 gifts that would mean the most to them. For adult family members, draw names and set a price limit, instead of everyone buying everyone gifts. Children in the family can do the same thing. For friends, agree on cards; it's the friendship that's the true gift.

Stress #3 Family: I love my family, and I'm sure you do too, but that doesn't mean they don't know how to push our buttons. Who are the challenging people in your family? Can you limit your time with them? When you do spend time with them, can you bring someone along who acts as a buffer? Make an escape plan. When you find yourself getting upset, plan to change the topic or leave the room. Can you take a walk? Can you go make a phone call to someone who will calm you down? Can you find a quiet room in the house and just breathe deeply? Do you need to manufacture an emergency and go home? Some families are more intense than others. Do what you need to do to take care of yourself.

Boost #1 Nutrient-Density: When life gets busier and more stressful, what we eat becomes even more important because it provides us with the nutrition we need to manage the stress. You can add AIP treats to your diet, but eat them alongside the best meat and seafood you can afford, lots of fresh vegetables, fermented foods, bone broth, and organ meats (the most nutrient-dense food of all).

Boost #2 Sleep: Sleep is directly related to inflammation in the body. Too little, and your inflammatory genes switch on, and your immune system goes into defensive mode. Prioritize getting 8–10 hours of sleep every night.

Boost #3 Schedule Joy: Sometimes we get so caught up in the obligations of the holiday season that we forget this is supposed to be a joyful time of year. Schedule one thing every week that will revitalize you. Maybe it's a pedicure or a pick-up game of basketball. Maybe it's a snowball fight or a tea date with a friend. Don't make this optional. Write it in pen on your calendar, and make these plans with people who light you up and leave you feeling better after their company.

Boost #4 Take a Daily Break: You can find 15 minutes somewhere. Is it in the morning before anyone else is awake? Is it right after the kids go to school? Is it your lunch break at work? Can you take 15 minutes when you get home, before facing whatever needs to be done that night? How about the 15 minutes before bed? Whatever you choose, commit to giving yourself this time every day, and temporarily turn off all contact with the outside world. Find a room where you can be alone in your home, or go outside. You can just be quiet and breathe. If that makes you nervous, do something relaxing: take a bath, go for a walk, listen to soothing music, or lie down for a little while. The important thing is to feel that this time is 100% yours and yours alone. This isn't selfishness. This is renewal.

The Most Important Tip of All: Forgive yourself. We're human beings, and sometimes we make mistakes. If you fall off the AIP diet train, forgive yourself and get right back on. Don't use it as an excuse to binge the whole season. It's much easier to recover from a day of indulgence than from a month. Keep an eye on the big picture: your health is worth more than any temptation you face this season.

CHAPTER 16

OVERCOMING SELF-SABOTAGE

So, you've learned which foods ramp up inflammation and which ones tone it down, and you're ready to get started. You're smart and your body lets you know when you stray, so it's easy to stick 100% to this protocol. Or is it? Changing habits, healing our bodies, and even making choices about food are all very complex, and there's not just physiology to address but psychology as well.

The truth is, sometimes we sabotage ourselves. Even knowing that a food is going to cause an autoimmune flare and result in pain or disability, we sometimes eat it anyway. Why is that? The answer is *not* simple, but I'm going to share some possibilities and provide you with tools to hopefully avoid this pattern altogether, or stop it if it's already part of your life.

First, let's look at some potential biological causes behind self-sabotage behavior. Inflammation can make us seek comfort through food, and we get trapped in a vicious cycle of increasing inflammation. Certain pathogenic bacteria in our digestive tracts prefer sugar and refined carbohydrates as food, and they affect our cravings. The more we eat those foods, the more we want them. Also, if we indulge in sugar or excess carbohydrates (like grains), it causes blood sugar imbalances that cause even more cravings. Vitamin deficiencies can also affect brain function, and so can brain fog—both of which are common symptoms of autoimmune disease. What does all this mean? When you first start the AIP, it's not unusual to have all of these forces at work causing physical cravings. The good news is that if you can power through and stick with the protocol 100%, your body will change. Your inflammation will reduce, your blood sugar will balance, your brain fog will clear, gut pathogens will die off, being replaced by beneficial bacteria instead. And if you focus on nutrient-density, you will resolve your vitamin deficiencies and improve your brain function to support good decisions in your life overall. This means that your cravings will reduce over time, sometimes going away altogether.

But it's not as simple as just biology. There are emotional triggers behind self-sabotage patterns as well, and they require more self-reflection to address. Feeling deprived often leads to feeling rebellious, even when we're the ones setting the rules. If we lack meaning and purpose in life, we can feel "empty" and respond by trying to fill that hole with food. Childhood issues can manifest as self-sabotage behavior. Negative thoughts and beliefs often lead to negative choices. Feeling betrayed by our bodies can make us want to "punish" them. Fear of change can also be a root of self-sabotage, even fear of wellness if we've been sick a long time. Lastly, sometimes we choose "fitting in" over taking care of ourselves. Healing diets are well outside of the mainstream, and our friends and family often tempt us to go off diet. I believe all of us can relate to at least some of these triggers, and some of us will find all of them familiar. What do we do about them? Even if you're not a writer, a journal can be a powerful thing. Explore some of these questions by writing about them and see what answers come forth. You can also talk about these issues with a good friend, or better yet, a therapist. Sometimes just bringing these triggers into the light—out of the unconscious and into our awareness—allows us to stop in that moment of emotion and make a different choice. Research even shows that simply naming an emotion removes some of its power over us.

Aside from sticking with the protocol until the physical cravings pass, and becoming aware of your own emotional triggers, what else can you can do to break the pattern of self-sabotage in your life (which often embraces far more than just choices around food)? Here are eleven tools for self-love and self-care which can help you overcome self-sabotage:

1. **Write a list of activities that soothe you,** which you can choose to do instead of eating unhealthy foods (or making unhealthy lifestyle choices). Post this list where you'll see it every day.

2. **Create a vision board**—a collage that represents what you want from your life. How do you want to feel? What abilities do you want to regain? What activities do you want to be able to do again? Look at this board every day, to set the stage for healthy choices.

3. **Get tested for gut dysbiosis.** If you have pathogenic overgrowths, you can often treat them with herbal antibiotics much faster than diet alone. The Paleo Mom Consulting can guide you through this process: Thepaleomomconsulting.com.

4. **Make sure you eat plenty of fat and protein** throughout the day, to keep your blood sugar balanced.

5. **In addition to a written journal, a dream journal or an art therapy journal can also help you** understand yourself better. It's also a great thing to do when you have a self-sabotage impulse. It gives you something else to do in that moment.

6. **Pay attention to your thoughts and beliefs,** and work to change negative perceptions into positive ones. This is called mindfulness. Often our self-talk is cruel, and we speak to ourselves in a way we would never speak to another person. When you hear yourself being critical, take a few deep breaths and say something loving or affirming to yourself instead.

7. **Find a support system for making healthy choices.** Pay attention to who among your friends and family acts in supportive ways, and spend more time with those people. In Chapter 17, I share my best advice for developing this support system.

8. **Practice assertiveness when being pressured by someone else** to make a choice that will hurt your body.

The more comfortable we are with our choices, the less other people challenge those choices.

9. **Have you ever heard of the Emotional Freedom Technique (EFT)?** It's a simple mind-body technique that can help you get past a self-sabotage impulse. It combines tapping certain points of the body with verbal affirmations. It might seem silly the first time you do it, but it's amazingly effective. I have a tutorial on my blog: Phoenixhelix.com/and-more.

10. **Learn your habit tendency.** In the book, *Better Than Before,* author Gretchen Rubin describes a theory called The Four Tendencies—that we all fall into one of four "habit personalities" and by knowing which we are, we can choose health strategies that work for us. I hosted a podcast on how this applies to the AIP. You can listen to it here: http://bit.ly/habitpodcast.

11. **Forgive yourself for your mistakes.** This is the ultimate act of self-love. If you do "slip up," get right back on the AIP wagon. Don't use it as an excuse to keep making harmful choices. It's much easier to recover from one mistake than many, and you deserve to feel good and to heal.

CHAPTER 17
GETTING SUPPORT

Reversing autoimmune disease through diet and lifestyle is something no one can do for us. We're the ones who decide the food we eat, what time we go to bed, how hard we push ourselves, whether we take time to de-stress. Yet, we don't walk this world alone. We're surrounded by friends, family and co-workers who are powerful influences on our lives. It's a lot easier to stay on the healing path if we're supported by those people, rather than thwarted by them. So, how do we get that support? Here are my best tips:

1. **Value your health enough to ask for what you need:** When it comes to reversing autoimmune disease, it's time to put yourself first. This is an unnatural feeling for a lot of people. We're used to taking care of others, often at the expense of ourselves. With autoimmune disease, our bodies are in crisis, and we need to do everything we can to heal ourselves. This is a time for self-love and self-advocacy, not self-sacrifice.

2. **Start with your home:** If at all possible, have your household kitchen match your healing diet. Chapter 9 gives

detailed instructions for creating an AIP kitchen. You may think this is unreasonable to ask of your family, but it's not. Autoimmune disease has a powerful impact on the family, as well as the person who is sick. Your healing benefits everyone. Terry Wahls' research reveals that the people who live in households that contain only diet-compliant foods succeed at a much higher rate than those who don't.

3. **Out of sight out of mind:** This doesn't mean everyone in your family has to eat identically to you. Family members can eat as they wish outside of your presence; just ask that they avoid eating "forbidden" foods in front of you.

4. **Serve delicious food:** The resource section of this book contains links to recipe archives online, as well as many wonderful cookbooks. The AIP is primarily well-prepared meats and vegetables. It's not weird-looking or weird-tasting food. Once your family realizes how delicious this food can taste, they're much less likely to object to eating it for dinner. For more tips, go to the Podcast section of my blog and listen to the episode, "Transitioning Your Family to Paleo": Phoenixhelix.com/media.

5. **Navigating change with friends:** It's very common for people to socialize with friends over food, so a change in diet actually changes the nature of your friendship. You may not be comfortable eating in restaurants often, and "happy hour" might be anything but happy if you can no

longer have the peanuts and beer. The first step is to have an honest conversation. Explain how your autoimmune disease makes you feel and how this diet has the potential to make you feel infinitely better. If your friends love you, they'll want you to heal. Tell them that their support means a lot. Try hard not to proselytize; often we're a mirror to the people in our lives, whether we intend to be or not, and they think we're judging their choices. Explain that this is about you, not them, and you aren't going to try to change them. Lastly, come up with new ways to spend time together. Go for walks, meet for tea, go to a play, attend an art show, or invite them to your house for a meal, a movie, or a game of cards. There are lots of ways to spend time with those we love without being surrounded by foods we can't eat.

6. **Let your healing speak for you:** If people aren't supportive in the beginning, they often become supportive when they see the improvement in your health. Let's face it, people are skeptical at first of this whole paleo idea. While it's logical that diet and lifestyle have a huge impact on our health, that's not what the TV commercials are selling, and culturally it's not how we were raised. When I told my mother my plans to reverse rheumatoid arthritis with diet, she actually laughed out loud. She thought I was crazy. But when she saw that it worked, she became 100% supportive. Now when I visit her, we

cook AIP meals for the whole family. The same thing can happen with your family and friends, so if your improvements aren't visible, be sure to talk about them with the people in your life.

7. **Be consistent:** People will only take your diet as seriously as you do. If someone offers you an inflammatory food and says, "Here, have a bite. A little bit won't hurt you," and you eat it, they are going to keep tempting you. Why? Because you've just shown by your actions that your diet is flexible. This is the hard part: walking the healing path when there are people in your life who aren't yet 100% supportive. Gather all the self-discipline at your disposal to say no. If you can avoid these people, do, and spend time with those who are encouraging your choices instead.

8. **Make new friends:** If there's no one in your life who is supportive, it's essential that you find that support elsewhere. Thankfully, there is a global community at your fingertips. If you're on Facebook, join the AIP Support Group. Otherwise, check out Thepaleomomcommunity.proboards.com. Lastly, if you live in one of the larger cities, there are local meet-up groups where you can find people who eat just like you. Autoimmune-Paleo.com posts a Community Update once a month, which includes lists of meetup groups around the world.

9. **The workplace:** Bringing your own food for lunch takes care of your daily needs, but occasionally there are work dinners or meetings with extra challenges. For the dinners, see if you can help organize them, picking a restaurant or catering company you trust. If you're going to be tempted by doughnuts at a meeting, keep some paleo-friendly snacks on hand just for you. Ideally, your work should be about your contributions rather than your diet. Still, people might have questions. Often, it's easier to keep the answers general: "I'm on a prescribed diet for health reasons." Only people who are truly interested will ask more questions, and it's up to you how much you decide to share.

CHAPTER 18

WHAT ARE CIRCADIAN RHYTHMS?

Circadian Rhythms affect all aspects of health, from hormone balance, to metabolism, to our ability to sleep well at night, and most important of all—our ability to heal. What are they? Simply put, they are our bodies' internal clock—the complex mechanism that lets our brain know when it's daytime and when it's night. You might think that would be obvious, and in ancestral times it was. In our distant past, we spent our days outdoors exposed to both sunrise and sunset, and there was no electricity to trick out bodies into thinking days last forever. Modern life has turned our circadian rhythms upside down. We spend our time indoors, exposed to constant blue light that mimics sunshine both day and night. And then we're surprised when we have trouble falling asleep or sleeping deeply.

How does this affect autoimmune disease? There are lots of factors, but let's start with sleep. Sarah Ballantyne recommends we get 8–9 hours of sleep every single night. Before you say, "I can't do that!" consider this: It's only recently that we've been getting less, mostly due to the time we spend on the computer and watching TV (both of which emit blue light, contributing to our sleep problems in two ways).

Why is sleep so important? It's when our body repairs itself. If we are trying to heal, we need to give our bodies the time and tools they need to do the job. Studies show that lack of sleep increases inflammation and puts the immune system into a defensive mode— pretty much a recipe for autoimmunity. And while we think we can "catch up on sleep" with a few extra hours here and there, it doesn't work that way. While we might *feel* more rested, the genes controlling inflammation remain turned on. Consistently getting 8–9 hours of sleep every night is what's needed to turn those genes off.

Many people suffer from insomnia. The first step to curing it is correcting your circadian rhythms—giving your body the cues it needs to recognize day from night:

- Get outside during the day and expose your body to natural light. Doing this first thing in the morning is ideal. Even 15 minutes helps.
- Work, socialize, exercise and eat your larger meals during the day. This is when we're meant to be active.
- Eat your last meal at least a few hours before bed.
- Limit your screen time in the evening, turning off TV, phones and computers a few hours before bed. If you can't do that, try wearing amber glasses to block out the stimulation of the blue light. There's also free software available that turns your computer screen amber at sunset, from Justgetflux.com.

- Start preparing for bed an hour before bedtime. Do something relaxing to wind down—read a book, take a bath, visit with your family, meditate, etc.

- Get on a regular sleep schedule. Our bodies like routine, and adults benefit from bed times and wake times, just like children do.

- Make your bedroom a sleep sanctuary. Don't allow phones or televisions in your room. Keep your room a comfortable temperature. Use a white noise machine to block out external sounds and blackout curtains as needed to block out external light.

- If pain keeps you awake at night, using pillows as bolsters can help. Hug one to support your shoulders, and place another either under or between your knees to take the pressure off your back and hips.

- If you have trouble falling asleep and staying asleep, don't stress about it. That makes the problem worse. Instead, follow the steps above and know that it will improve with time. In the meantime, rest in bed—even if you aren't sleeping. That's still beneficial. If you must get up, keep your screens turned off and do something relaxing until you can fall back asleep.

Our circadian rhythms aren't just about sleep. They're about overall health. I said in the beginning of this chapter that these rhythms also govern hormone balance and metabolism. Hormones directly affect autoimmune symptoms, which is why so many women are diagnosed with autoimmune disease after a big hormone shift, like menopause or having a baby. It's also why some women experience increased symptoms around their menstrual cycle. Those are sex hormones, but other hormones affect autoimmunity as well, like cortisol—the stress hormone. When it goes out of balance, people often suffer from adrenal fatigue, where they feel bone tired during the day but "wired" and unable to sleep at night. Balancing our circadian rhythms helps balance all our hormones, thereby easing our autoimmune symptoms (instead of exacerbating them).

CHAPTER 19

GENTLE DETOXIFICATION

We live in a world where we are assaulted daily by pollution in our air and water, chemicals in everything from food to furniture, and plastic so abundant it now shows up in our bloodstream. Our bodies have natural detoxification pathways, but they are overwhelmed by modern life. More than 80,000 new chemicals have been released into the world since the industrial revolution 150 years ago, and most of them within the past 50 years. These chemicals have never been fully tested for their effects on our bodies or the environment. We are asking our bodies to detoxify far more than they were designed to handle.

So, how can we boost our detox capability? The first step is to limit the amount of toxins entering our bodies by looking closely at the products we buy. The second step is to gently increase our body's ability to clear itself of the toxins we've already accumulated. Thankfully, the autoimmune protocol gives us a head-start. Back in Chapter 6, I mentioned that organ meats have 10–100 times the nutrition of muscle meats, and those nutrients help our bodies detoxify. That's one of the reasons they are such an important part of this diet. Additionally, vegetables support this process, too—

especially sulfur-rich vegetables like cauliflower, kale, onions, garlic, mushrooms, cabbage, broccoli and asparagus. Terry Wahls recommends we eat 3 cups of vegetables from that category every day.

We don't recommend detox supplements or chelation protocols on the AIP. There are two phases of liver detoxification. The first phase liberates the toxin, and the second phase deactivates it. Many people have difficulty with phase two. If toxins are liberated but not deactivated and excreted, they're actually more dangerous than when they were stored inertly in your body. That's why many people feel sick on aggressive detox protocols. You are essentially getting poisoned with your own released toxins. It's much better to detoxify slowly, at a pace your body can handle. A nutrient-dense AIP diet helps internally, and here are three gentle supports you can apply externally that also assist this process:

- **Epsom Salt Baths:** Not only are these baths relaxing and wonderful for stress reduction, they also increase sulfate in the body similarly to eating sulfur-rich vegetables. There is no hard and fast rule on the amount of Epsom salt to add to the bath. Start with one cup and see how your body responds. If it knocks you flat, use less the next time. If it wasn't relaxing at all, use more.

- **Dry Skin Brushing:** This simple technique increases flow of blood and lymph throughout the body. Our lymphatic system runs right alongside our blood circulation. Where the blood brings nutrition to every cell, the lymphatic system helps clean up the toxins leftover from cellular processes and illness recovery. Use a long-handled, natural fiber, firm-bristle brush. Gently run the brush over your entire body, always brushing in the direction of your heart. An ideal time to do this is before you shower.

- **Saunas:** Sweating is another potent detox pathway, effective at removing heavy metals, solvents and plastics from our bodies. Saunas are a great way of sweating at a much higher rate than we can achieve any other way. It's one of Terry Wahls' favorite detox protocols. That said, some autoimmune conditions have a symptom of heat intolerance. If that's you, wait until that symptom has cleared and approach sauna therapy slowly. Terry herself used to have that symptom but now tolerates saunas very well.

So, those are ways we can remove toxins that are already in our bodies, but how can we reduce our toxin exposure in the first place? Look at the products you are buying and using in your home, both beauty and hygiene products, as well as cleaning products. Many of them contain the harmful chemicals mentioned in the introduction to this chapter. An excellent online resource to healthy shopping choices is The Environmental Working Group. They research chemical safety closely and recommend the best choices: EWG.org.

However, we don't even need all of the products we buy. We've just been convinced by marketing companies that we do. Personally, I clean my entire house with vinegar, baking soda and a mild natural dish soap. Those are the only cleaning supplies I own. I've also cut way back on my beauty and hygiene products. I've switched to the oil cleansing method for my face—search online for instructions. I use Primal Pit Paste for my deodorant, which is simply coconut oil, baking soda and lavender essential oil. And I brush my teeth with baking soda. My body thanks me for all of these changes.

Pay attention to big purchases as well. For example, modern furniture is filled with chemicals like flame retardants and formaldehyde. Antiques (or used furniture) are safer choices because they've had a chance to off-gas already. If you are painting or remodeling your home, choose low-VOC paints and stains and choose environmentally safe building materials. Fill your house with plants—they are natural air filters, and open your windows regularly to ventilate. Consider a water filter as well, especially if you live in a community that chlorinates the water. Did you know that most water supplies carry residues of prescription medications—everything from birth control hormones to ibuprofen? A reverse osmosis filter is the one type that removes these pharmaceuticals. Lastly, limit the amount of plastic in your life. At the very least, don't ever cook or heat things up in plastic (or nonstick pans)—that causes a transfer of plastic particles into your food.

CHAPTER 20

STRESS REDUCTION

Stress! Its importance relating to health has been in the headlines for decades. We experience stress every day in healthy doses and some days (maybe most days) in unhealthy amounts. Even so, we're often in denial about its impact on our lives. The truth is, stress impacts autoimmune disease just as much—if not more—than diet. You can't ignore this fact and heal. There's a whole field of science called psychoneuro-immunology. It's a big word, but it simply means that our thoughts and emotions impact our immune system. It sounds new-age, but it's actually science. There's a great book by Donna Jackson Nakazawa called *The Last Best Cure*. In it, she shares the details behind the science, but she also conducts a personal experiment. Over the course of a year, she adds mindfulness meditation, yoga and acupuncture to her life, and then tracks their impact on her autoimmune symptoms. The results are dramatic. I encourage you to do a similar self-experiment. Here are 10 ways to reduce stress. Incorporate some of these techniques into your life every single day:

1. **Sitting Meditation:** This idea intimidates a lot of people. We imagine monks sitting still for hours with quiet minds,

compared to us trying to sit still with crazy-loud minds. We think we are not like the monks. The truth is, if you're human you think, and even monks have thoughts during meditation. The key is to avoid following the thoughts. Simply notice them and let them pass. There are a few tricks to make this easier. One is to focus on the breath and fill your mind with that awareness. Another is to say a mantra. Om is a classic one, and it means "the sound of the universe." But you can also focus on the words Love or Health or Peace. While sitting in silence can be soothing to some, you can also listen to soft music while you meditate. And a wonderful beginner's method to meditation is guided visualization. There are many such CDs sold on Amazon.com as well as free videos on YouTube.

2. **Moving Meditation:** You don't have to sit still to experience the benefits of meditation. Yoga, tai chi and qi gong are all forms of moving meditation, where you become aware of your body, your breath, and the energy that flows through you. You can even practice walking meditation. Go outside and walk slowly, opening up your senses. Feel the ground under your feet, the feeling of your feet as they step onto and off the ground, the sounds that surround you, the sunshine (or moonlight) above, the feeling of the wind across your skin. Then turn your senses inward. Gradually scan all parts of your body: your ankles, shins, calves, knees, thighs, hips,

pelvis, back, chest, shoulders, arms, neck and head. When you become aware of tension anywhere in the body, let it go.

3. **Mindfulness—Presence:** Most of the time we aren't "here now." Our thoughts fill our awareness, and we spend most of the time in the past or the future: worrying, planning, obsessing, remembering, and stress comes from that. Mindfulness is simply the practice of tuning into the present moment. You can make any activity mindful. Here are two examples: (1) Mindful Eating: Sit at the dinner table with no distraction (no television, no book, no smartphone and no conversation). Instead, take a deep breath, relax your body, and focus purely on the food you are eating. What's the texture and taste? How does it feel on your tongue? Pay attention to every bite. It can be a blissful experience. (2) Mindful Dishes: We do a lot of dishes on a healing diet. This is a way to enjoy that process. Again—no distractions. Immerse yourself into the experience. Feel the warm water wash over your hands. Watch the dishes as they become clean. Are there patterns in the water? Do the dishes sparkle? Is there steam? It's surprising—but there's beauty everywhere when we are truly present.

4. **Take a Computer-Free Day:** Have you noticed that your attention span is really short lately? That you can't sit still, you lack focus, you bore easily, you feel anx-

ious all the time, and are easily irritated? These are all direct effects of constant intermittent use of the computer throughout the day and night. This includes smartphones, tablets and desktops. Partly it's how we use them—in small time fragments every few minutes throughout the day. Partly it's the blue light they emit at night that's over-stimulating to our brains and bodies, which we already talked about in the chapter on Circadian Rhythms. See if you can go 24 hours with no computer use whatsoever. If that feels overwhelming, start with 8 hours. Here's a tip: keep a notebook nearby and when you feel a compulsion to send an email, post to social media, or research something on the internet, write it down. You can do it tomorrow. As the hours pass, those compulsions pass too, and a deep relaxation sets in that you likely haven't felt in a very long time. That deep sense of peace is incredibly healing, and it's amazing to realize that just a few decades ago in our computer-free past, we felt that way most of the time.

5. **Get Outside Some Place Beautiful:** In modern life, it's easy to forget that human beings evolved to live outdoors, and we miss it! Scientific studies show that spending time in nature not only lowers stress chemicals in the body, it also alleviates depression, improves attention span and strengthens the immune system.

6. **Get Creative:** Art isn't just for artists and children. We

all have creativity within us, and giving ourselves time to express it can be both relaxing and rejuvenating. It can be as simple as enjoying an adult coloring book or keeping a mandala journal. You can take your camera outside for an hour and photograph whatever strikes your eye. Or do something formal like take a painting or sculpture class. And there are many expressions of art beyond the visual: music, dance, writing, poetry, theater—even cooking can be an art form if we allow ourselves to play and enjoy the process. Whether you pursue this informally or formally, find an outlet that frees your own soul.

7. **Learn to Say No:** This is essential to stress reduction because there are only so many hours in the day, and if you have autoimmune disease, you often have limited energy reserves. Add to that a healing diet and lifestyle which requires a greater time commitment for both cooking and sleeping, something has to give. Saying no feels unnatural to some people, and if that's you, it's time to practice. Take a good look at your life and see what responsibilities you can let go and transfer to someone else. If you don't think you can let anything go, consult an objective friend to help you prioritize.

8. **Byron Katie's The Work:** Sometimes we really struggle with letting go of negative thoughts. We quiet them for a while, but then they return with a vengeance. Byron

Katie has a simple method for turning these thoughts on their head. She calls it "The Work," and it involves questioning your thoughts and seeing if their opposite is equally true. This may come as a shock, but there is always an opposite truth, and once you see it, the negative thought loses its power over you. Here's a quote from Katie: *"You don't have to believe everything your thoughts tell you. Just become familiar with the particular thoughts you use to deprive yourself of happiness. It may seem strange at first to get to know yourself in this way, but becoming familiar with your stressful thoughts will show you the way home to everything you need."* For more information, visit Thework.com.

9. **Professional Care:** In *The Last Best Cure*, the majority of the stress reduction techniques the author implemented were self-driven, but she did add professional acupuncture toward the end of her year-long experiment, and she loved it. She felt like it put her into a meditative state immediately. If you can afford it, treat yourself to some professional self-care to help you relax. Acupuncture is one, but there are many other forms of bodywork: massage therapy, lymph drainage therapy, craniosacral therapy, reiki, myofascial release, etc., and they can all promote healing. Also, there's a time and place for psychological counseling as well. Living with autoimmune disease is stressful in itself, and research

studies also show that many people with autoimmune disease had difficult childhoods. Dr. Datis Kharrazian, a leader in the field of autoimmune disease, says that healing cannot happen if we don't face our emotional demons. In fact, we often stay busy to avoid facing them, so it's not uncommon to feel them rise to the surface when we take time to be still and relax.

10. **Keep a Gratitude Journal:** When life is difficult, we often focus on the negative and miss the positives altogether, but this creates a biased, untrue view of life. There is beauty all around us, even when we're struggling, and noticing that beauty restores some of the joy we've been missing. A gratitude journal is a practice of looking beyond ourselves. Every day, write down three things for which you're grateful. Here's the catch: be specific and try and choose something different every day. Sarah Ban Breathnach, author of the book *Simple Abundance*, says: *"We think it's the big moments that define our lives—the promotion, the new baby, the renovated kitchen, the wedding. But the narrative of our lives is written in the small, the simple, the common. The overlooked. The discarded. The reclaimed."* So, pay attention to the small gifts of daily life. It might be your child's laugh, or a hummingbird at the window, a recipe that turned out perfectly, a phone call with an old friend, a smile from a stranger, a rainbow on the way to work,

discovering a new favorite TV show, a flower blooming in your garden, or the silence after a winter snowfall. Each time you notice and appreciate something positive in your life, you send a healthy cascade of chemical reactions through your body. Gratitude is medicine.

CHAPTER 21

HOW TO SURVIVE AN AUTOIMMUNE FLARE

For those of us living with autoimmune disease, there's no scarier word than "flare." It brings up pain, disability, fatigue and fear. A major motivation for doing something as challenging as the AIP is to eliminate flares from our lives. However, healing through diet and lifestyle takes time. It's not an overnight "fix." So, what do you do if you flare during this process?

- **Don't let a flare define your world.** Having a flare doesn't mean you're not healing. And flares don't last forever, even though we fear they will.

- **Make yourself a priority.** This is a time to take care of yourself. If you're used to taking care of others and also have a busy life, you might be in the habit of putting yourself last. During a flare, you need to put yourself first. Cancel any optional obligations, and ask your loved ones for help.

- **Relieve your pain.** For many autoimmune diseases, a flare means intense pain. Don't feel any guilt about relieving it with medication. Although many of us have the goal to get off our meds, that takes time too. It's not healthy to suffer with pain.

- **Sleep.** For many autoimmune diseases, a flare means intense fatigue. For all human beings, sleep is when the body heals and regenerates. Go to bed early, sleep in late, take naps. I know that sometimes the symptoms of a flare can make sleep difficult. Prop yourself with pillows for greater comfort, and just do your best to rest, any way you can manage it.

- **Focus on healing foods.** While it's good to always focus on nutrient-density with the AIP, it's especially important during a flare. Drink lots of bone broth, eat organ meat and seafood. Homemade soups are especially nourishing during this time.

- **Drink ginger tea between meals.** It's a natural anti-inflammatory and digestive aid. Grate or mince some fresh ginger root (about a teaspoonful) into your mug and pour some boiling water over it, cover, and leave for 3–5 minutes. Pour through a small sieve and add optional raw honey to taste.

- **Don't binge.** During a flare, it's easy to think, "Screw it! I feel awful anyway, I'm going to do whatever I want." And then you binge on bad food, which unfortunately amplifies and lengthens the flare. It may be called comfort food, but it really should be called pain-inducing food. You deserve better. Choose healing foods that provide the real comfort instead.

- **Detoxify.** Health is a constant balance of nourishment and detoxification, and during a flare, you need support in both areas. Try one of the gentle methods described in Chapter 19.

- **Cry.** I remember once when I was fighting back tears, a wise woman said to me, "Tears are healing, so don't fight them. Let them flow." It's true. Grief is part of the process.

- **Laugh.** This sounds counter-intuitive, doesn't it? How can you laugh when you feel awful? But this is the time you need to laugh the most. It's a natural stress reliever and anti-inflammatory. Famed author, Norman Cousins, treated his ankylosing spondylitis through laughter therapy, saying it was the best pain relief he could find. So watch a funny movie or TV show, trusting that it's medicine.

- **Practice self-love.** During flares, we can get very angry with our bodies, feeling like they're attacking. But our bodies are doing the best they can to heal, and they need our love in these moments more than ever. Read Chapter 22 to see that your body is not your enemy.

- **Meditate.** You may think that meditation is impossible during a flare, but for me, it was essential. There's the physical reality of a flare, which is intense, but strong emotions can make a flare even worse. I would get angry and full of rage. I would get terrified that it would never stop. My heart would race, and the inflammation in my body would ramp up. That's the opposite of what I needed. Meditation didn't take away my physical pain, but it calmed me down and restored a feeling of emotional and mental peace, which are healing emotions. Meditation isn't just for the masters, and even 15 minutes can do wonders. In Chapter 20, I share many different ways to reduce stress.

- **Journal.** Sometimes we need to express our emotions before we can let them go, and journaling is a wonderful way to do that. If you're not a writer, keep a sketch journal. Art therapy is equally powerful.

- **Music therapy.** We've all been moved by music. Some songs make us want to dance, others make us cry, others make us simply stop and listen because they're so beautiful. During a flare, the type of music that soothes you might be soft, like a caress. Or it might be a loud song that does the screaming for you. Choose whatever music speaks to your soul.

- **Hug therapy.** Hugging releases oxytocin, which is a hormone that calms the body down and makes us feel good. And it works whether it's your spouse, your child, your sister, your friend, or your pet. There's even a study that says hugging yourself can reduce pain. So, fill up on hugs. There's no limit.

- **Sunshine medicine.** If the weather is nice, lie in the sun. Its warmth soothes, being outdoors refreshes, and the Vitamin D you get from the sun's rays helps the body heal.

- **Harness the mind-body connection.** When you're in a flare, it's natural to obsess on it, but doing so can make the flare worse. If you have identified the cause of the flare, it's also easy to fall into the trap of replaying the scene in your mind, wishing it had never happened. But the brain is interesting—each time you replay a scene, it's like it's happening again in the present moment. This can lengthen a flare, which you absolutely don't want. So, instead, any time you find yourself obsessing, take a deep breath and visualize the flare in your past, not your present. Then visualize something that makes you happy, and focus on that instead. This can take practice, but the more you do it, the more you'll notice when you're obsessing, and the easier it becomes to replace that obsession with a positive image.

- **This too shall pass.** Remember that flares are temporary. When you're in the midst of one, it's easy to forget. I feared every flare I had wouldn't stop, even though flares, by design, are temporary. So, fight that fear by saying the mantra, "This too shall pass," over and over until the fear is gone.

- **Surrender.** We have such negative associations with this word. We think it means giving up. In reality, it simply means letting go. When I would flare, I would tense up (of course) and would feel myself fighting to try to make the flare go away. This had the opposite effect every time. It was like my flare fought back. Surrender can feel very peaceful. It's simply accepting the present moment. Surrender can be a gateway through a flare.

CHAPTER 22

YOUR BODY IS
NOT YOUR ENEMY

Words are powerful. I learned that as a little girl, the first time someone made me cry on the playground by saying they didn't want to be my friend. I also learned the power of positive words: accepting compliments without rejecting them (it took practice), and as a young woman in the midst of first love, experiencing the fear and the bliss of saying "I love you" for the very first time and hearing those words in return.

I'm a writer and an avid reader. Words are my joy and my outlet. But some words I reject, specifically the ones the medical establishment assigns to autoimmune disease:

- Your body is attacking you.
- Your immune system is out of control.
- Your body is broken.
- Your body has betrayed you.
- You will continue to get worse.

Can you feel your heart start to race reading those statements? They're terrifying. I have a different perspective. My body wants to heal and is doing everything in its power to do so. Autoimmunity is a miscommunication within the body, not an intentional war within. Symptoms are my body's way of telling me something's wrong and asking for help. I had many signals for many years before rheumatoid arthritis hit. Like many people, I misinterpreted or ignored those signals.

Here's a fact: My body does a million things right every day, which I take for granted. From a steady heartbeat and oxygen supply, to trillions of cells doing zillions of processes every second, sending signals bodywide that let me move my fingers to type these words, allowing me to speak, to sleep, to sing and to love, controlling all aspects of homeostasis from body temperature to cell regeneration, my body is amazing and is totally on my side.

- **My body needs my love, not my anger.**
- My body's potential is infinite.
- My body and I are one. There is no separation.

This isn't a Pollyana viewpoint. It's *hard* having an autoimmune disease. Even though many of us speak of the gifts that come with life's challenges, let's be honest: we'd much rather be 100% healthy. Some days, we need to cry. Other times, we want to scream. Even though I have reversed the course of my rheumatoid arthritis and am 95% better, I have a very sensitive body that requires vigilance, and I miss feeling free. But I don't hate my body. I don't blame my body.

Every day I re-commit to loving my body, and I believe that's essential to healing. If your child is sick, do you get mad at them, or do you nurture them and do everything in your power to help them be well? Don't our bodies deserve that same unconditional love? Don't we?

CHAPTER 23

KEEPING A SYMPTOM JOURNAL

It's a fact of human nature that we tend to notice what's wrong, more than we notice what's right. When something gets better, we often forget it was ever a problem. This is especially true when improvements happen slowly. The way to notice (and celebrate) these improvements is by keeping a symptom journal—two actually. One is a daily journal where you write down a quick summary of how you're feeling. The other is a monthly journal where you review your daily notes and summarize. Looking back at where you started and seeing how far you've come is very empowering and worth a few minutes of your time each day.

Journals can also show healing plateaus or setbacks, which can be motivation for re-evaluating your diet and lifestyle choices—where do you have everything dialed in, and where can you still improve? Often it's the lifestyle piece that we let slide, yet it's just as important as diet. I also go over some troubleshooting steps in Chapter 26 if you're doing the AIP perfectly and still not seeing the results you seek.

What to Include in a Daily Symptom Tracking Journal

- **Sleep quality:** Did you fall asleep easily or did you have insomnia? How many hours did you sleep? Did you wake often or sleep deeply? Did any muscle cramps or pain wake you?

- **Waking state:** Did you wake feeling refreshed or did you feel groggy? Any morning stiffness? If yes, what level and how long did it last?

- **Pain:** Rate your pain on a scale of 0–5, and document where in your body you are feeling it.

- **Mental state:** Are you experiencing brain fog, or is your mind clear? How is your memory? Concentration?

- **Emotional state:** Are you happy, sad, angry, depressed, numb? Is your mood stable or swinging from one state to another?

- **Medication:** If you are on any PRN medications (meaning that you take them only as needed), write down when you need them and what dose. If you are on daily prescribed medication, your need for these might change as you heal. Work with your doctor to see if you can reduce or eliminate these safely. The ability to do this varies based on the individual, and purpose of the medication.

- **Energy levels:** Do you get tired during the day? Do you need a nap? Do you feel caffeine-dependent? Are you hyperactive? Or is your energy strong and balanced throughout the day?
- **Exercise:** Are you able to exercise? If yes, what form did you do today and for how long?
- **Digestive state:** Any bloating? Indigestion? Constipation? Diarrhea? Discomfort?
- **Skin condition:** Any increase or decrease in rashes, acne, psoriasis or eczema? Is your skin drier than usual or starting to glow with health?
- **Dietary changes:** Did you start any new supplements? Did you eat out at a restaurant (often a source of hidden ingredients)? Have you started reintroductions (described in Chapter 24)?
- **Lifestyle:** Did you meditate? Take time to relax? Do something that brought you joy? Take a bath? Get outside? Endure a stressful situation?
- **Detox:** Have you implemented any of the measures discussed in Chapter 19 to remove toxins from your body or your lifestyle?
- **Mark the day:** Keep track of how long you've been on the AIP. It's empowering to see yourself pass markers like 30 days, 6 months, 1 year. Note: strict AIP isn't meant to last forever. Once you have seen a clear reduction in your

autoimmune symptoms, you can start the reintroduction process described in Chapter 24. This is how you personalize the AIP for you.

Monthly Summary

- At the end of the month, summarize how you felt and see how it compares to prior months.
- You can use a notebook and keep this journal by hand, or use any word processing program. There are also free websites like Chartmyself.com, if you prefer to do it online, and Symple is a free app for the iPhone.

REINTRODUCING FOODS

Strict AIP isn't meant to last forever. This is a healing diet, but it contains two distinct phases: elimination and reintroduction. The first phase we've already discussed in detail: we eliminate the foods that are potential inflammation triggers. Now we get to the fun part: reintroductions! Once you have seen a clear improvement in your autoimmune symptoms, you have a baseline for reintroducing foods back into your diet. This isn't permission to go back to the way you were eating before AIP. I need to be honest with you—that's unlikely to happen. However, you *can* expand your diet again, and there's a very specific process for figuring out which foods benefit your body, and which foods are your personal inflammation triggers. That's important to understand—we're all different—and the reintroduction process lets you personalize the AIP for you.

When can I start? The minimum time to wait is 30 days. Some people wait longer—anywhere from a few months to a year. There are three things to consider when making this decision: (1) You don't need to have achieved complete remission, but you do need to have seen clear improvement in your autoimmune symptoms. This gives you a baseline that allows you to interpret food reactions during the reintroduction process. (2) Sarah Ballantyne believes that the longer you do the elimination phase of the AIP, the more your body has a chance to heal, and the more successful you will be with reintroductions. Terry Wahls disagrees—she worries that being on an elimination diet long-term can lead to nutrient deficiencies that can become their own obstacle to healing. They're both right. You don't want to rush into reintroductions before you're ready, but you don't want to stay on the elimination phase of the AIP forever either. Safely expanding your diet is the goal. (3) Emotions play a role. If you are afraid of the reintroduction process, you need to wait until you're ready, because fear can cause flares just as much as food does. Conversely, if you are feeling emotionally overwhelmed by the elimination phase of the AIP, you'll want to begin reintroductions as soon as possible. Feelings of anger and sadness and frustration that sometimes accompany food restrictions can cause flares and interfere with healing too. Your decision about when to start reintroductions should take both your physical and emotional wellbeing into account.

What's the process?

- Choose one food to reintroduce at a time.
- Take a series of tiny bites which minimize the risk of intense reactions. Start with 1/2 teaspoon and wait 15 minutes. If you have no reaction, eat a full teaspoon and wait another 15 minutes. If no reaction, eat 1–1/2 teaspoons. then wait a few hours.
- If you had no reaction to the tiny bites, go ahead and eat a normal size portion of that food. Now stop eating

the food altogether, and watch your body for symptoms over the next 3 days. Reactions can happen anywhere from immediately, to a full 72 hours later. A reaction is an increase in your autoimmune disease symptoms. This might be pain, fatigue, difficulty sleeping, a skin rash, digestive distress, brain fog, moodiness, etc.

- If you have a negative reaction, you know you are intolerant and should avoid that food. Wait for the symptoms to pass before reintroducing another food, so you have a clear baseline for each reintroduction.

- If you had no reaction at all (or such a mild one it's hard to tell if the food was the cause), then it's time for the second phase of the reintroduction process. Eat a little bit of this food every day for a week, and monitor your body again. Food intolerance seems to come in two forms. (1) A strong reaction, where there's no doubt that your body reacts negatively to the food. (2) A cumulative inflammatory response that starts off so mild you can miss it at first, but becomes noticeable after daily consumption. If after eating the food for a week, your body still feels good, then you know that food is not a problem, and you can introduce the next one.

Tips regarding interpreting food reactions: As human beings, our bodies fluctuate from day to day; some days we feel a little better than others, and some days we feel a little worse. When you're monitoring for a reaction, you're looking for a clear response outside of the range of your normal fluctuations. Emotions can also affect the reintroduction process in two ways: (1) Denial: you reintroduce a food, have a negative reaction, and think to yourself, "There's no way this is a food reaction; it's gotta be something else." That's one of the reasons there's a second phase, where you eat a little bit of the new food every day for a week. If the food causes a reaction, there will be no question by the end of the week. (2) Fear: you're so afraid of what might happen when you reintroduce a food that the emotion itself causes you to flare. Emotions are powerful; don't ignore them. Practice the stress reduction steps in Chapter 20 throughout the reintroduction process.

Strength of food reactions: Sometimes a food reaction is mild, but other times it's intense—more intense than prior to the AIP. Why is that? When you eat a food regularly, to which you are intolerant, your body goes into a chronic state of inflammation in response. Symptoms vary from person to person. It might be digestive distress or joint pain or mood swings. For people with autoimmune disease, it exaggerates the symptoms of your disease. When you eliminate this food for 30 days or more, two things happen: (1) You start to feel better, and (2) your body has a chance to calm down its defenses. Then, when you reintroduce the food, the response can be acute. Although it feels bad, this is actually a good thing because you have a clear communication that this food harms your body. As long as you stop eating the food, the acute response goes away, and you return to feeling better than ever before.

Which foods do I reintroduce first? You choose a category of food, and reintroduce the least potentially allergenic food in that category and slowly work your way up to the most allergenic:

- **Introduce egg yolks by themselves, before introducing whole eggs.** Most people tolerate the yolks well. If there's an intolerance, it's usually to the egg white. Note: Soy is a common chicken feed, and research shows the soy protein is transferred to the eggs. If you find you're intolerant to eggs, you might actually be reacting to the soy. Some people have found that they can eat pastured soy-free eggs, but not conventional ones, for this reason.

- **Introduce seeds before nuts.** (1) Start with fruit-based spices (like black pepper) and seed-based spices (like mustard and cumin). (2) Next, test seed-based oils (like sesame). (3) If that went well, proceed to soaked and dehydrated seeds, (4) Then try seed butters and flours, raw seeds and toasted seeds. (5) Finally, test cocoa and coffee separately. Although they're seeds, the body responds to them uniquely. The best way to reintroduce cocoa is through homemade chocolates, so you isolate other variables. (Store-bought chocolate often contains soy and refined sugars.) The same goes for coffee. Don't go to Starbucks; make it at home. (6) If you digest most seeds well, you're ready to try nuts. Start with the nut oils (like walnut and macadamia). (7) Then try soaked and dehydrated nuts. (8) Then try nut butters and flours, raw nuts and toasted nuts. Why? Seeds are easier to digest than nuts, and soaking seeds and nuts increases their digestibility another level. Individual vs. group: Since many people find they tolerate one type of nut or seed and not another, it's best to reintroduce one variety at a time. Tip: When you're ready to try toasted seeds or nuts, it's better to buy them raw and toast them at home, rather than buy toasted ones from the store. Store-bought varieties are often toasted in refined oils not allowed on the paleo diet (such as canola oil).

- **For dairy, reintroduce in this order:** (1) grass-fed ghee, (2) grass-fed butter, (3) raw goat yogurt or kefir, (4) raw goat milk, (5) raw goat cheese, (6) raw cow cream (7) raw cow yogurt or kefir, (8) raw cow milk, (9) raw cow cheese. Why? Dairy is made of three components: butterfat, lactose and casein. Many people don't have a problem with butterfat, which is why ghee and butter come first. If there is a food intolerance, it will usually be to the lactose or the casein (milk is highest in lactose and cheese is highest in casein). Raw dairy is recommended as long as you can find a trusted source. It contains living enzymes that make it easier to digest, as well as a higher nutritional profile. Lastly, goat dairy is introduced before cow dairy, because goat dairy is easier to digest.

- **Introduce fresh legumes before dried legumes.** While green beans and peas are technically legumes, they are easier to digest than the dried varieties. Many people tolerate them well. Dried legumes, on the other hand, aren't officially part of the paleo diet, and many people never try to reintroduce them. However, there are a growing number of people who believe they are good food for our beneficial bacteria (if tolerated). If you choose to reintroduce, you will want to soak or sprout them before cooking, to enhance their digestibility.

- **White rice—the "preferred grain."** This is the one grain that many people embrace in the ancestral health community. Why? In conventional nutrition, white rice is considered the worst choice because unless it's enriched, it doesn't have much going for it nutritionally. That's because the hull has been removed from white rice, which contains the "nutrition." It turns out that's also the reason it's embraced by some corners of the paleo community. The hull also contains the anti-nutrients—those food components that interfere with digestion and nutrient absorption, exacerbating our guts and causing an inflammatory response. Since those anti-nutrients have been removed, many people consider white rice to be a harmless grain. However, like all foods, some of us tolerate it and some of us don't. If you choose to reintroduce, cook it in bone broth and a healthy fat, for added nutrition, and eat it alongside a meal to moderate the blood sugar impact.

- **Nightshades are recommended as the last reintroduction.** This is because they are one of the most common food intolerances for people with autoimmune disease, and the effects of the inflammation after reintroduction can take longer to tone down. When you reintroduce them, do so one vegetable or spice at a time. While some people find they are intolerant to all nightshades, others find they tolerate some and not others. A list of nightshades is included in Chapter 5.

- **Foods we don't reintroduce:** The goal with the AIP reintroduction process is to expand our diet with healthy foods that our body tolerates well. We don't reintroduce foods that we know are harmful—like wheat, gluten, sugar, food additives, inflammatory refined oils, etc. Living well with autoimmune disease means feeding our bodies well for life. After the food reintroduction process, most people find their diet fits somewhere between paleo and AIP. We call that Personalized AIP.

Tips for reintroduction success: This is science, and you are the experiment. It's a careful process where you pay close attention, control the variables, and listen to what your body tells you. It's also incredibly empowering. Once you learn to communicate with your body like this, it's a skill you have for life. The first thing to do is take notes. In the prior chapter, I taught you how to keep a symptom journal. That's helpful any time, but it's essential during the reintroduction process. Second, cultivate patience. This process takes many months to complete, but it's worth the effort. I've written a detailed guide that includes a lot more tips as well as recipes for the reintroduction process: http://bit.ly/reintroductions.

CHAPTER 25

TOP 5 MISTAKES PEOPLE MAKE ON THE AIP

A lot of us learn through trial and error. The beauty of starting a protocol that thousands of others have done before you is that you can learn from other people's mistakes and get it right on your first try!

MISTAKE #1: NOT COMMITTING 100%

In the paleo movement, people talk a lot about paleo perfectionism and how it's better to follow the 80/20 rule, to take the pressure off and make the lifestyle sustainable. This means you follow the rules 80% of the time, and break them when needed. If you're following paleo for weight loss or to tweak some minor health issues, this might work. Unfortunately, if you have an autoimmune disease, it doesn't. We have to follow the 100% rule, and I get it: that sucks. It's a lot of pressure, but the stakes are high and the rewards worth it. We're trying to do what the doctors say is impossible. We're reversing disease that took years to develop in our bodies. We're literally transforming our genes. That's no small thing, and that's why we need to be "all in." Marriages with only 80% commitment don't make it. Parents would never be only partially committed to their children. You are an amazing human being and worth a 100% commitment to yourself and your health.

MISTAKE #2: IGNORING NUTRIENT DENSITY

Healing diets focus a lot on removing foods that promote inflammation and exacerbate autoimmune disease. And it's true that avoiding these foods is essential to healing. Our immune systems will stay overactive if continually triggered by food intolerances. However, there's another side to this equation, and that's the healing power of nourishing food. I focused on this in Chapter 6 of this book, but it bears repeating. We need rich and diverse nutrition for our bodies to rebuild on a cellular level. There are specific foods that help this process: organ meats, wild-caught seafood, bone broth, healthy fats, and lots of fresh vegetables. A diet of chicken breasts and AIP-friendly desserts isn't going to get you there.

MISTAKE #3: RUSHING THE REINTRODUCTION PROCESS

The AIP is hard to do. It's restrictive and time consuming. For that reason, many people force themselves through the elimination period (barely) and then binge on all the restricted foods at once. Unfortunately, this nullifies the whole experiment. Remember why you're doing this: you want to heal, and the AIP is a powerful healing tool when done correctly. It allows your body to communicate very clearly about the foods that are helpful vs. foods that are harmful. However, this communication happens during the reintroduction process. If you rush it, you not only miss that valuable information, but you have to go back and do the elimination period all over again. No one wants to do that! Follow the tips in Chapter 24 on how to do reintroductions correctly. It is absolutely the key to developing the personalized diet that is right for you.

MISTAKE #4: THINKING IT'S JUST ABOUT THE FOOD

Diet is a huge component in healing, but it's not the only one. That's why I have chapters in this book that focus on the importance of sleep, stress reduction and learning to befriend your body. Negative thought spirals and unhealthy lifestyle patterns can cause autoimmune flares just as powerfully as food, if not more so. The AIP is a holistic approach to healing. Be sure to address it from all sides.

MISTAKE #5: NOT GETTING THE SUPPORT YOU NEED

This is a tough one. Some of us are lucky enough to have people in our lives who are completely supportive of our healing journey. It's much easier to stay on a healing diet if your family joins you (or at least doesn't tempt you by bringing home pizza for dinner). The same goes for friends; many people have talked about so-called friends sabotaging their efforts, which can make your already difficult life, much harder.

I really don't think you can do this alone, so that means finding the support you need to succeed. One way is to have the tough conversations with your friends and family which will hopefully get them on board. If not, reach out to others who are on the same journey. I've dedicated Chapter 17 to all the steps you can take to develop your personal human safety net.

CHAPTER 26

TROUBLESHOOTING

The first thing to know is that the AIP isn't a quick fix. It took time for autoimmune disease to develop in your body, and it takes time to reverse that process. If you have a flare after starting the AIP, it doesn't mean it's not working. Your flares (and other symptoms) should reduce in number and intensity, but that happens over many months, not overnight. Hopefully, they will go away altogether. That said, the healing journey is about progress, not perfection. So use the symptom journal I describe in Chapter 23, so you can celebrate each improvement.

This chapter presents some solutions to problems that might develop unexpectedly when you first transition to the AIP, as well as troubleshooting if the AIP doesn't give you the results you seek.

Digestive Issues

Most people's digestion improves on the AIP because foods are removed that interfere with digestion and irritate our digestive tract. However, sometimes the damage that's been done to our bodies over the years leaves us with impaired digestive abilities, and we might need some extra support. If you are experiencing gas, bloating, constipation or diarrhea, here are some steps that might help:

1. **Relax while you eat.** Digestion actually starts in the brain. We have divisions in our nervous system to take care of different functions of our body. The unconscious processes like digestion need our parasympathetic nervous system, in order to function. That's the relaxation nervous system. So, sit at a table when you eat. Take a few deep breaths, relax your shoulders, chew slowly, and really enjoy your food. Don't watch TV, text, read a book or surf the internet. Be present. You'll be surprised by what a difference this can make.

2. **Boost your stomach acid.** In spite of the antacid ads on TV, most people don't have enough stomach acid, and that's what leads to indigestion (which people then treat with antacids, making the problem worse). We need stomach acid to digest our food, which allows it to release from the stomach into the small intestine where other digestive enzymes are triggered to release like dominos. If we don't have enough stomach acid, all of our digestion is impaired. We can naturally boost our stomach acid by chewing on a piece of raw ginger before or after our meals, eating sauerkraut alongside our meals, or drinking a tablespoon of apple cider vinegar in a very small glass of water after our meals. Start implementing one or all of these tips and see if you notice improvement.

3. **Watch your posture when you eat.** Are you slouched in a chair or hunched over the table? If so, you're compressing your digestive organs. That makes it hard for them to do their job. Instead, take a deep relaxing breath, and sit up straight. I noticed an immediate improvement in my digestion when I started paying attention to my posture.

Weight Concerns

Depending on your autoimmune disease, you might be worried about weighing too much or weighing too little. Both are normal side effects of our illness, and as we heal on the AIP, our weight often corrects itself.

It's important that we don't prioritize weight over wellness. In our culture, we tend to be obsessed with body size, and I've seen people try to count calories on the AIP in an effort to lose weight, but that cuts their nutrition, and we need nutrition to heal. I've also seen people try to force-feed themselves past satiety in an effort to gain weight and only make themselves sicker. The best thing to do is to eat a moderate amount of food, eating plenty of each macronutrient (fat, protein and carbohydrate), and focus on nutrient-density by following the AIP food pyramid in Chapter 6. If you're not sure what's moderate, Cronometer.com is a free website that tracks not only calories but nutrients as well. Enter your daily food intake for a week and see how you're doing. A good average goal is 2,000 calories, containing high amounts of a wide variety of micronutrients.

That said, there are two other things that also affect our weight: sleep and stress. If we don't get enough sleep and don't reduce our stress, our hormones will always be out of balance and interfere with our ability to achieve not only a healthy weight, but health in general.

When to Get Help From a Professional

The autoimmune protocol appeals to self-starters, people who are good at self-care, self-discipline and self-analysis. It can be hard for us to ask for help. We feel like we "should" be able to figure it out ourselves. But autoimmune disease is complex. Healing is a lifelong journey, and it often has many layers. Health coaches, nutritionists, functional medicine practitioners, and medical doctors can all offer expertise that we simply don't have. If you hit a healing plateau of a few months or longer, that's a good time to seek outside help.

There are many factors that might be interfering with your healing. Here are some possibilities, and they all require professional help to test, diagnose and treat:

- Gut dysbiosis
- Parasites
- Small intestine bacterial overgrowth
- Co-infections
- Hormone imbalance
- Chemical intolerance
- Nutrient malabsorption
- Vitamin deficiencies
- Gut-brain axis problems

- Brain inflammation
- Adrenal fatigue
- Misdiagnosis, or a missed diagnosis
- Autoimmune activity that requires intervention in addition to diet and lifestyle.

There's a wide variety of skill level among functional medicine practitioners. In the next chapter (AIP Resources), I'll share some recommendations. Always look for someone who understands the paleo diet and also someone who can prioritize. You shouldn't have to spend thousands of dollars to be assessed, nor should you leave the office with a sack full of supplements. Interventions work best one at a time, or, at most, a few at a time. A qualified professional should be able to guide you regarding where to troubleshoot first.

CHAPTER 27

AIP RESOURCES

My Blog

Every week, I share free information on my blog to support your AIP journey. There's a weekly recipe sharing event, called the Paleo AIP Recipe Roundtable, giving you new ideas so you're never bored in the kitchen. My archives page of past roundtables includes over 1,500 AIP-friendly recipes. I also write articles related to autoimmune healing, sometimes sharing personal experiences, other times sharing new research or tips for healing. And I have a blog store that contains every AIP resource currently available: Phoenixhelix.com.

My Podcast

I love podcasts, both as a listener and a host. Mine focuses 100% on reversing autoimmune disease through the paleo diet and lifestyle. I combine interviews with professionals and authors, with interviews with people like us who share their experiences with autoimmune healing. It's a great way to get information easily while doing other things, like driving to and from work, or doing household chores at home. You can find me on iTunes or Stitcher: Phoenix Helix.

Functional Medicine Practitioners

- The Paleo Mom Consulting is a team of professionals who are experts at both the AIP and troubleshooting for autoimmune disease. The team includes health coaches, nutritionists and functional medicine practitioners: Thepaleomomconsulting.com.

- There are also two websites that list medical doctors and alternative health practitioners who believe in the paleo template to healing: Primaldocs.com and Paleophysiciansnetwork.com.

- And there's a small but growing number of autoimmune specialist MDs who are open to the paleo approach as a complementary treatment to medicine: http://bit.ly/paleomds.

Peer Support

- It's much easier to do the AIP when you're not doing it alone. There are online support groups where you can find others doing the AIP too. Facebook has two active ones: AIP Support Group and Autoimmune Paleo Recipes. If you're not on Facebook, try Thepaleomomcommunity.proboards.com.

- I'm hoping after reading this book, you feel ready to embark on the AIP and be successful. If you still feel nervous, I recommend an online group coaching class called SAD to AIP in SIX. The program guides you from the Standard American Diet to the Paleo Autoimmune Protocol over a 6-week time period. Some of my friends who are health coaches lead the classes, and 20 other people are in the group with you. You get peer and professional support all at once: http://bit.ly/aipclass.

AIP Books, Cookbooks, Meal Plans, Convenience Foods, Cooking Ingredients and More

There are so many wonderful resources that make life on the AIP easier. I've gathered all of them together for you in one place in my blog's Healing Store. I also add new ones as they become available, so you always have the latest tools and foods at your disposal: Phoenixhelix.com/store.

GRATITUDE

I would like to say thank you to some special people who helped make my recovery (and therefore this book) possible:

- The original AIP posse: Mickey, Angie, Whitney and Christina. I'm so happy you're my tribe.
- The growing AIP blogger community, with whom I share laughter, questions, answers and collaboration. This would be a lonely road without you.
- The scientists who did the research upon which the AIP is based and the educators who made the information public. While I can't name everyone, I would like to especially thank Sarah Ballantyne, Terry Wahls, Robb Wolf, Loren Cordain, Datis Kharrazian, Boyd Eaton and Staffan Lindeberg.
- My husband for supporting me from day one on this journey and being my partner in food, love and life.
- My family for loving me enough to worry about me in the beginning, and then believe in me when they saw my health turn around.
- My friends and family who have cooked me AIP meals. There is no greater gift.
- My blog readers and podcast listeners, who give me daily encouragement for my own healing journey and inspiration to continue spreading AIP knowledge to the world. You are my community!

ABOUT THE AUTHOR

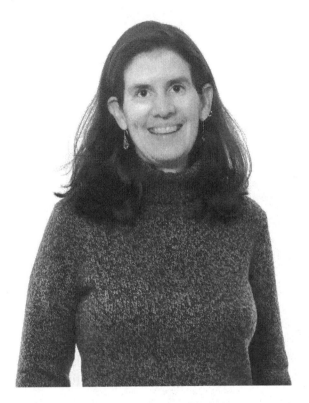

Eileen Laird uses the paleo AIP diet and lifestyle to manage rheumatoid arthritis. Her popular blog, Phoenix Helix, receives 1 million unique visitors annually. She features recipes, research and personal stories about the autoimmune experience. She also writes Autoimmune Answers, a regular column in *Paleo Magazine*, and is the host of the Phoenix Helix Podcast, the only paleo podcast focused 100% on autoimmune healing.

Made in the USA
San Bernardino,
CA

58926455R00082